CW00661744

Understanding

A practical guide to managing your symptoms

Dr. Susan Avery

Copyright © 2020 Stephen and Susan Avery

All rights reserved. No part of this book may be reproduced or used in any manner without written permission of the copyright owner except for the use of quotations in a book review.

ISBN 9798642190432

For more information, email
info@beatthemenopause.com

Contents

Introduction

One fine autumn day in 2012 I found myself lying down in the middle of the afternoon because I had no energy to do anything. I ached all over as if I had the flu, but there were no other flu symptoms. Even thinking was beyond me, and that was why it took so long to figure out what was wrong. I was 53 years old, and my periods were appearing at random. I had been having hot flushes, little tidal waves of heat that swept through me from time to time, but not the severe night sweats that some women experience. Nevertheless, all the signs were telling me that I was due to be a victim of that great hormonal conspiracy known as the menopause - but no one told me that I would be transformed from a fairly fit, active, alert, happy human into a lifeless wreck almost overnight. This was not supposed to happen to me. There is an idea floating about that your experience of the menopause is likely to echo that of your mother. My mother barely noticed it (but then my mother is of a cheerful stoic disposition, and even gave birth with very little fuss). Sadly, I have not inherited her physiology, or her disposition.

The good thing about all this, was that, having had the revelation that it was my aging endocrine system that had laid me low, I made a rapid recovery with the aid of a sympathetic GP and some HRT. I was my old self within a fortnight, energy levels back to normal and hot flushes banished.

Talking to middle aged female friends and acquaintances I discovered that my experience was not typical. In fact, there does not seem to be a typical experience of going through the peri-menopause, into the menopause and beyond.

Physical symptoms vary, so do the emotional manifestations, and, of course, medical advice can be very different depending on which school of thought your family doctor subscribes to….

These last can vary from: -

"quick take these pills"

through

"try natural oestrogen and acupuncture"

to

"it's all perfectly natural, pull yourself together and don't make such a fuss…."

And then there is the minefield that is the internet…..

Here you can find all manner of advice from the "washing your hands in a silver salver at midnight under a full moon" variety, to how to buy hormones on the grey market, to the story of the woman who ran three marathons, wrote her first novel and learned to juggle, in spite of night sweats and mood swings.

As women we undergo two major hormonal upheavals in our lives. These are associated with the arrival and departure of menstruation or periods. Periods are a damn nuisance. However, their arrival signals the beginning of the reproductive phase of our lives, just as their departure signifies the end. Puberty wasn't exactly a barrel of laughs. There were so many physical changes to adapt to. Our bodies changed shape, we sprouted hair in unexpected places, we had spots - spots are not just part of teenage identity, but the result of changes in the levels of androgens, usually referred to as male hormones, but just as vital for female physiology and development. Then, of course, there were the expectations and aspirations, mostly unrealistic, and mostly unfulfilled that lead to the endemic teenage state referred to by parents as "moping around" or "sulking". Of course, we knew we were in a poetic state of melancholy, which should probably be best indulged in in a garret in Paris or St Petersburg. All this would be interrupted once a month by something messy, and for many of us, downright painful (not to mention being preceded by mood changes that, depending on your temperament, might involve homicidal tendencies, or the urge to jump off Beachy Head).

Puberty was no fun. But we survived, and with any luck, came to terms with our plight and our raging hormones, which would slowly settle down.

At the other end of the road, instead of being delighted to see the end of this monthly ritual, many women dread its departure like the impending loss of a dear friend.

Confirmation that our reproductive lives are over is a source of distress for some. In reality any possibility of unassisted conception fades out up to ten years before we experience the full force of the menopause. Nevertheless, for some women, the disappearance of the menstrual cycle seems to signal the arrival of old age.

This is, of course, nonsense.

The menopause is not a monster lurking in the bushes, preying on middle aged women, turning them into shriveled wrecks overnight.

The menopause is not a cliff that we tumble over to find we are suddenly old and no longer capable of doing all the things we enjoy.

It isn't something to be afraid of - just something to be aware of, and to be prepared for so that you can recognise any problems or challenges when they occur.

The menopause is a natural process. It is not sudden. Changes occur over a long period and you may not notice any real changes for some time.

There's no question that some of us experience unpleasant, uncomfortable symptoms, but these don't last forever, and these days we have choices as to how we treat or manage them.

On the other hand, some women have no symptoms at all, and slide painlessly from one phase of their lives to the next.

Symptoms or not, there are changes to the way our bodies function, and understanding these can help us deal with any problems that do arise – and understanding how our lifestyle and behavior influences our health beyond middle age, can have a real impact on the quality of our later lives.

I have a background (and a career) in reproductive science and medicine, so I have more knowledge than most of female anatomy and the action of our hormones. But as a female going through the menopause I struggled to find a comprehensive, clear and friendly resource to help answer my questions.

In 2017, BBC Radio Sheffield carried out a survey of over a thousand women in their 50s and 60s, and only 28% considered that they had a strong understanding of the menopause prior to experiencing it, and only 32% felt that their GP was helpful. Information about the menopause online or in print has a tendency to be depressing, alarming and sometimes baffling.

There is plenty of advice to be had about HRT, dietary supplements, natural remedies, and lifestyle changes, but it isn't always easy to pick out what is real, unbiased, appropriate and helpful for you as an individual. We are all different, and, aside from our physical differences, we may have very different emotional responses to the changes in our physiology. We may also have philosophical or religious views about the use of medication to relieve menopausal symptoms.

What is important is to find a way to deal with your symptoms rather than let them control you.

In this book I have tried to distill, from the plethora of information available, the facts and ideas that are likely to be most useful and interesting. I hope to help the reader understand what the menopause is, and how to live through it in the least traumatic way. Above all I intend to show that the menopause is not an illness, and that, like most of life's problems, it can be dealt with by taking a calm and practical approach based on facts and not mythology.

Chapter 1 - What is the Menopause?

The menopause is not an illness....say this to yourself loudly and emphatically, even when you are in the midst of a hot flush. It is a consequence of living through our forties into our fifties, and infinitely preferable to the alternative.

The word has its root in the Greek mens, meaning month, and simply refers to the cessation of monthly periods. Some might think of it as the end of the reproductive phase of our lives, but in truth our chances of pregnancy are close to zero ten years before we are fully menopausal. Fertility declines from puberty onwards, with the rate of decline increasing from around the age of 35, and taking a nosedive as we hit our forties. However, the ovaries continue to function as endocrine glands (glands that produce hormones) after they cease to produce eggs, but this function also declines over time. Then our periods become irregular, and bleeding may be heavier or barely noticeable, last for longer than usual, or only a day or two. Finally, they stop completely. At this point we are considered menopausal. Until this point we are considered to be peri-menopausal - on the brink of the menopause. Our hormone levels may indicate that we are peri-menopausal as long as ten years before our periods cease.

On average the menopause sets in between the ages of 45 and 55, although about one in a hundred women are menopausal before the age of 40. The precise age of the menopause may be influenced by a number of factors. Your genes play a significant role. Daughters of women who had an early menopause have a high chance of following in their footsteps. Evidence of stress and the environment as factors is emerging. A study published in November 2019 of nearly 2000 women across Europe, shows that women who live close to green spaces have lower levels of the stress hormone cortisol. Lower cortisol has a positive influence on oestrogen levels, and, as a result, the menopause may be delayed by eighteen months on average.

These days women can expect several decades of life of reasonable quality, bearing in mind the general ageing process, after the menopause. Human females are unusual in having three phases to their lives – pre-puberty, the reproductive phase from puberty to the peri-menopause, and a post reproductive phase, the menopause. In most species females continue to reproduce throughout their lives.

There has been a great deal of speculation about the evolutionary role of this post-reproductive phase. It occurs in two other mammalian species, the killer whale and the short-finned pilot whale, but we are unique among primates. Given that the main purpose of existence for any species is to reproduce, it seems odd that human females live such a considerable proportion of their lives in a state where they are apparently useless in biological terms. Human males may continue to produce offspring into old age, but human females just stop.

This lack of understanding has contributed to the negative view of the menopause and that phase of life which follows it. Biologically it seems that post-menopausal women have no purpose. This has, in the past, lead to a view that women in later life were really just a burden on society, being of no use whatever, as they could not reproduce and were no longer sexually attractive (the only other possible justification for female existence). This is a very western view. In other societies, the role of older women is better established, especially in matriarchal societies. They are respected for their experience and play a significant part in holding the family structure together.

In the west our view of femininity is heavily bound up in appearance and reproductive potential. We invest a great deal of resources in staving off the effects of ageing which would probably amuse our counterparts in other parts of the world.

The role of older women in the family structure may give us a clue to the reason why human females have such a long, post reproductive phase to our lives.

In societies where reproduction is allowed to take place naturally, women will have their first child around the age of 19, and their last at 39. As a result, the one generation ceases to produce offspring as the next starts.

In killer whales, the offspring of older mothers have much lower survival rates compared with offspring of their daughters. It makes sense for them to stop producing offspring with high mortality rates, and invest their energy in their grandchildren. There may come a point where supporting the upbringing of your offspring is more effective in perpetuating your genes than continuing to produce your own. Competition for resources is likely to favour the younger parents and their offspring, so it may be better to focus on being a grandparent.

This hypothesis may be a good fit for killer whales, but it may simply be a hypothesis of convenience for humans, a partial fit but not a full explanation. The risk of congenital abnormalities in humans increases with maternal age, as the supply of normal, fertile eggs runs down, but this is just a feature of the programmed limit on our reproductive lifespan. It is by no means certain which question needs answering – "why do we stop reproducing so early in our lifespan", or "why do we live so long once our reproductive term runs out?"

One other possible reason why the "grandmother" hypothesis might fit is the comparative helplessness of human infants for the first decade of their lives. It might be that to successfully raise a large brood of human infants requires the support of a willing grandparent who has finished producing her own offspring.

Whatever the precise evolutionary reason for our post reproductive survival, the huge changes in social structures, particularly in the West, mean that these considerations are irrelevant for vast numbers of women, as the extended family becomes increasingly rare.

In any case, we do have to deal with the physiological effects of the menopause. Understanding the nature of the changes our bodies undergo, should make it easier to cope with the symptoms. It should also make it easier to separate fact from myth.

It all begins with hormones..

A little bit about Hormones.....

Hormones are blamed for all sorts of human quirks and ills. Teenage sulks are bound to be due to hormones. A disagreeable female must be under the influence of hormones.

In fact, all our bodily functions are driven or influenced in some way by hormones.

School biology teaches us that hormones are the body's messengers. They are produced by various glands in response to different triggers - changes in the external environment, changes in the internal environment, emotional responses. They signal other organs to respond (sometimes by producing other hormones in a kind of messenger relay). The word hormone comes from the Greek, meaning fire starter, and they are responsible for igniting the bodies responses to various triggers and conditions.

Why do changes in the way hormones are produced have such a dramatic effect on the way we feel and function?

The human body is a highly complex biochemical machine. Feeling fit and well depends on all organs functioning in equilibrium, and this, in turn, depends on communication. The nervous system and the endocrine system (hormones and the glands that produce them) form the lines of communication throughout our bodies. These lines are complicated. A small change in one element can affect entire systems dramatically.

Adrenalin is a hormone. If we have a shock or experience a sudden threat, signals from our nervous systems lead to adrenalin being released from the adrenal glands that sit just above the kidneys. Adrenalin is the hormone responsible for making sure we are fit for action. It begins a cascade of chemistry that affects our entire body. Our heart rate speeds up, our breathing gets faster, blood pressure rises, pupils dilate, blood is diverted to the muscles, and our metabolism is adjusted to maximise glucose levels to maintain energy levels in the brain. Legend has it that soldiers on the battlefield have lost limbs without feeling pain under the influence of adrenalin. Like adrenalin, many of our hormones have multiple, complex effects on our physiology which affect us both physically and mentally.

Whether we like it or not, we are our chemistry.

Which Hormones are involved in the Menopause?

Oestrogen is famously blamed for most of the negative effects of the menopause and there is no doubt that changes in Oestrogen levels have the most significant impact. It is involved in many aspects of physiology apart from reproduction (see figure 1), and this accounts for the wide-ranging symptoms of the menopause.

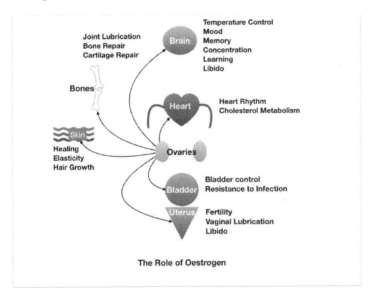

The Role of Oestrogen

The Oestrogen Roller Coaster

Oestradiol, the most significant form of oestrogen in human females, is mainly associated with the ovaries, and reproduction, but like adrenalin, changes in oestrogen levels affect the body in a number of ways. To give you an idea, excess oestrogen can cause acne, loss of libido, constipation and depression. These are distinct physiological effects - the depression cannot be attributed purely to the fact that you have acne, no libido and are constipated, even though this is enough to make anyone feel depressed.

Low levels also cause depression, fatigue and mood swings, as well as osteoporosis - a degeneration of the bone structure, leading to an increased risk of fracture.

Again, we can see that one hormone has a whole spectrum of effects, and the symptoms we associate with the menopause and with ageing in women, are those produced by low oestrogen.

Symptoms of the Menopause

Menopausal symptoms start to appear during the peri-menopausal phase. In a survey of just over a thousand menopausal women in the North of England, the symptoms that the majority considered to have the greatest impact on their lives, were hot flushes, night sweats, and difficulty sleeping. Mood swings come in just below these three, closely followed by problems with memory and concentration, joint aches and pains, anxiety, and a reduced sex drive.

Other symptoms that featured in the survey were vaginal dryness and discomfort during sex, headaches, palpitations, recurrent urinary tract infections, and menopausal acne, reflecting the wide-ranging role of oestrogen, and the impact of falling concentrations.

Hot flushes and mood swings have their own chapters, while other symptoms are dealt with below

Sleep and the Menopause

If you suffer from hot flushes and night sweats, and/or mood swings and anxiety, it is no wonder that you have disturbed sleep. Disturbed sleep is a consequence of other menopausal symptoms, not a discreet symptom in itself. Most of us will experience problems with sleeping at some time, whether short term, in relation to particular events, or illness, or longer term. During the peri-menopause, and the menopause proper, some women experience chronic sleep problems. Sleep disturbance or deprivation has a major impact on our ability to cope and function during our waking hours. Lack of sleep can also lead to depression and anxiety, which, in turn, may increase your problems sleeping.

Dealing with your menopausal symptoms should help to relieve your sleeping problems. However, this is easier said than done, and, in any case, the menopause is a really good cue for looking at your sleeping habits and what has become known as sleep hygiene. If you optimise your sleeping conditions, you may be able to reduce the impact of your menopausal symptoms.

Good Sleeping habits

Stopping watching any form of screen at least one hour before you go to bed – this includes phones and tablets as well as TVs and computer monitors. The blue light emitted by all of these devices can fool the brain into thinking it is daylight, and confuse your circadian rhythm. Sleep is mediated by a hormone called melatonin, the production of which is governed by changes in light. Daylight suppresses melatonin production, for obvious reasons, so dim light and darkness are important in helping us to achieve natural sleep.

Try reading, or listening to relaxing music in the hour before bed time – don't be tempted to get around this by taking melatonin pills – there is no real evidence that they work in the same way as physiologically produced melatonin.

Go to bed and get up at regular times-research has shown that regular sleeping hours may be more important than the number of hours you sleep when it comes to feeling rested and alert the next day. Regular hours reinforce your circadian rhythm, and help to facilitate regular patterns of melatonin production, which, in turn, will give you better sleep quality.

For the same reasons, try and avoid falling asleep before bedtime, and do not be tempted to hit the snooze button on your alarm on waking.

Keep your bedroom cool – no more than 67 degrees Fahrenheit or 19 degrees Celsius. Like fading light, a drop in temperature is important for melatonin production. A fall in body temperature is part of the process of initiating sleep. On the other hand, do make sure you are not too cold. It is difficult to sleep when your body is using energy to regulate your temperature because you are too hot or too cold.

Make sure your bed is comfortable and inviting. You need a comfortable, supportive mattress and pillows. Your duvet or blankets should not be in danger of sliding off during the night. Make sure you keep your bedding clean to avoid a build up of dust, dry skin and other potential allergens. Adjust your bedding as the whether changes in order to maintain a comfortable sleep temperature.

Regular exercise will also help you to sleep. On the other hand, you should avoid exercise within three hours of bed time. Exercise will raise your core body temperature, which will hinder sleep, as well as releasing stress hormones which will put your body on alert, and inhibit the production of melatonin.

Avoid coffee and other caffeinated drinks in afternoon and evening. Caffeine can stay in your system and affect your state of alertness for six hours or more.

Avoid drinking too much alcohol, and do not drink alcohol at all close to bedtime. Alcohol causes you to fall asleep more rapidly than usual. This may seem like a good thing, but alcohol has negative effects on sleep quality. Alcohol is a diuretic – in other words it increases the rate at which the kidneys produce urine. As a result, your bladder will fill faster, and you will need to get up more often in the night. You will also feel dehydrated, and drinking water will add to the problem.

Alcohol also affects your breathing by causing the muscles of your throat to relax. This leads to snoring and sleep apnoea, a condition where you may stop breathing or take only shallow breaths for anything from a few seconds to over a minute. This can cause you to wake, but even if you continue to sleep, you are more likely to suffer from fatigue, and longer term health problems.

Finally, alcohol reduces the amount of REM (Rapid Eye Movement) sleep, considered by many to be the most restorative form of sleep.

Try to avoid eating anything less than an hour before bedtime. Expending energy on digestion does not help with sleep, and lying down before your food is digested can lead to acid reflux and indigestion. If you eat a large meal in the evening, try and finish eating three hours before you go to bed. Eating may make you sleepy, but does not promote long or good quality sleep.

Have a bed time ritual that only includes actions that you associate with relaxation. This may include making a hot drink, or reading for a while (nothing too exciting, no adrenaline, please...), or listening to music on a timer so that it will switch off if you fall asleep. Anything you associate with sleeping and being relaxed will help.

What about milky drinks?

Milk contains tryptophan and melatonin. Melatonin, as discussed above, is a sleep mediating hormone, and tryptophan is a precursor of serotonin, a hormone which can also be converted into melatonin. You might reasonably expect that this combination would help you to get to sleep. Unfortunately, there is no evidence that melatonin taken by mouth can be assimilated into the system and have the same effect as naturally produced melatonin. The situation is the same with tryptophan.

If you do find that a hot milky drink does help you sleep, it is probably because this has formed part of your bedtime ritual for a long time, and you associate it with relaxation and sleep.

Depending on the type of drink it might also be an effect of magnesium. Malted milk drinks contain magnesium, which promotes the production of gamma–Amino butyric acid (GABA), a sleep promoting hormone. Magnesium is absorbed when you take it by mouth, so these drinks can have a sleep promoting effect via magnesium. On the other hand, be aware that these drinks may also contain high amounts of sugar, so they are not necessarily healthy.

If you are awake, anxious and restless in the night, the process of getting up and making a hot drink may help to relax you, and simply drinking something hot can divert blood from your anxious brain. Try Chamomile tea. Chamomile has been used for hundreds of years, as an herbal remedy for a whole range of conditions, but is probably best known for its supposed relaxing effects. It contains apigenin, which also promotes GABA production, although it is by no means certain that a cup of Chamomile has enough apigenin to have a real effect, as there are no conclusive trials. I drink Chamomile at bed time, and if I wake in the night, and find it helps with sleep, but this may just be the "hot drink" effect.

On the other hand, Chamomile does not contain anything nasty or fattening. Not everyone likes the taste, but adding honey can help.

Don't lie there and suffer...

If you can't sleep because you are too hot, or are feeling anxious, try getting up and moving around. Make a hot drink, sit and drink it somewhere comfortable, read a book for a few minutes. Go back to bed when you feel cooler/and or more relaxed.

If you lie in bed, worrying that you can't sleep, you will begin to associate bed with the stress and misery of sleeplessness. A change of scene and position can help to break this cycle.

Changes to Memory and Concentration

Some women report problems with memory and concentration as they move through the perimenopause into the menopause. This is affectionately known as "brain fog", and generally reduces or disappears after the menopause.

Is there really such a thing as Menopausal Brain Fog?

During the perimenopausal period, and the menopause proper, you may experience difficulty focusing, and you may find your capacity to learn new information is reduced, as well as experiencing difficulty with short term memory. Is this really caused by the menopause, or is it just part of aging?

Well, the good news is, for most of us these problems disappear by the time we are through the menopause, so clearly this is not purely age related. So what causes our brains to misbehave?

Aside from any specific cause, you should bear in mind that the menopause may bring a number of problems that can affect our cognitive ability, such as poor sleep, anxiety and mood swings. Learning and concentration are not easy when you've been awake half the night, suffering from hot flushes.

On top of this, the fluctuations in oestrogen that we experience during the perimenopause may have a direct effect. Oestrogen has multiple effects on brain function, on the transmission of signals between cells, on the generation of synapses, the junctions between brain cells, and on energy generation in the brain. Studies have been carried out on pre-menopausal women to investigate how brain function is affected by the menstrual cycle, and changes have been found in performance at times when oestrogen is high. It is also fair to say that the decline in oestrogen does play a part in brain aging, but generally the fluctuations in oestrogen during the peri-menopause seem to cause more problems than when oestrogen finally stabilises, even if it is at a lower level.

How can we combat Brain Fog?

To begin with we need to deal with the confounding factors such as lack of sleep. Practice good sleep hygiene (see above). Working on mood swings and anxiety will also have an effect on your ability to concentrate, which in turn will help with recall.

Give your brain a good work out regularly – crosswords, Sudoku, any sort of puzzle will help. Make an effort to focus – or learn a new skill, whether it is physical or intellectual. Reading also helps.

Aerobic exercise helps to boost oxygen levels, and circulation to the brain.

Eat a healthy diet – plenty of vegetables and fibre. A diet high in carbohydrates and fat will make you more sluggish.

HRT will help by replacing oestrogen.

Finally, don't let lapses of memory of concentration add to your anxiety. They may be frustrating, but they are common and not sinister, and they should ease and stabilise as your oestrogen levels settle.

Joint Aches and Pains

The cause of aches and pains during the peri-menopause and the menopause proper depend on the nature of the aches and pains. Some of us experience a kind of general ache, the sort of miserable feeling you would associate with extreme fatigue, or even flu. In fact, many women experience a feeling exactly like the muscle and joint aches associated with the flu, and this is because they have the same root cause. Our immune response to the flu involves the release of cytokines, chemicals that support the activity of our white blood cells in combating the flu virus. These cytokines have the unfortunate side effect of causing muscle and joint inflammation, resulting in aches and pains, sometimes severe. There is evidence that a decline in oestrogen levels triggers an increase in the same cytokines, leading to the same inflammatory response and the same aches and pains.

Taking HRT will relieve these symptoms fairly swiftly, but for those for whom HRT is not an option, or who would prefer not to take HRT, ultimately your body will adjust to the new lower levels of oestrogen, and the aches will pass. It is important to fight back as much as possible, and keep moving and exercising. Research has shown that even moderate exercise can have a significant effect on cytokine levels, and exercise, of course, has multiple benefits.

In the longer term, and more seriously, lack of oestrogen can result in an increased risk of osteoarthritis, as oestrogen is involved in the maintenance of cartilage, ligaments, and lubrication of the joints. Oestrogen is also involved in general bone health – see chapter 5, health after the menopause.

Again, HRT will help to reduce this risk. However, taking regular exercise, maintaining a healthy weight, and eating a healthy diet, as well as making sure you keep well hydrated, will al help to keep your joints healthier for longer.

Menopausal Acne

From our teenage years we are familiar with the idea that changes in hormone levels affect our skin. Ironically the shift in balance between oestrogen and testosterone that occurs at the menopause, may result in outbreaks of acne, especially on the chin, jaw, and around the mouth. Unlike teenage acne, the spots tend to be deep under the skin, and the large, red cysts of teenage acne do not occur. However, the basic cause is the same, pores that become blocked and inflamed as a result of excess sebum, the oily substance produced by the skin, under the influence of testosterone.

Menopausal acne is rarely severe, more of an irritation. It may begin in the lead up to the menopause, in the early stages of your hormonal changes, and will usually disappear once you are post-menopausal and your hormone levels settle down. If it causes you distress or discomfort, your doctor may prescribe either a cream or lotion, or occasionally antibiotics or other oral medication.

Avoid oil based cosmetics as they may add to, or even trigger the problem. Make sure you cleanse your skin with a product that does not dry the skin out (even though instinct might tell you that something astringent might help), and use a light moisturiser. Scrubbing your skin may help to spread the problem so treat it gently.

Naturally HRT will prevent the problem, or bring an end to it if it has developed before you start your HRT, but acne is not sufficient reason to take HRT if you do not wish to take it for any other reason.

The Menopause and your Sex Drive

The sex drive in humans is complex, involving all the senses, the brain and the imagination, as well as hormones and there are many factors that affect it. Drinking, smoking and obesity will all have a negative effect on our sex drive, as will stress and fatigue, and these factors may have a greater impact than the menopause.

Not all women experience a decrease in sex drive during the menopause, indeed, the fluctuations in hormones, and the changes in the ratio between oestrogen and testosterone can lead to an increase in libido. However, other symptoms of the peri-menopause and menopause proper could understandably cause you to have a reduced interest in sex. After all, poor sleep, hot flushes, and general aches and pains are not likely to have a positive impact on your interest in sex. Once your hormone levels have settled down, the lack of oestrogen has some specific effects, in particular a reduction in vaginal lubrication (see chapter 5). However, some women find the fact that sex is no longer connected with the risk of pregnancy liberating, and others find their appetite for sex increases, not only during the peri-menopause, but once they have passed through the menopause proper. Marie Stopes, the great campaigner on Women's health issues during the first half of the twentieth century, reported receiving letters from women in their 50s and 60s who were concerned that they still craved an active sex life. One woman, who, while going through the menopause had told her husband that their sex life was over, wondered how to tell him that, now she had gone through the change, she was desperate to resume normal activities.

We are all different, especially when it comes to sex, and the menopause affects us in different ways. There is no reason to assume that your libido will be wiped out by the menopause, or that the way you feel during the menopause will set the tone for the rest of your life.

There is a view that our sense of identity, and of being female, is inextricably bound up with our desire or need for sex (as opposed to how desirable we are to others). This puts pressure on those women for whom sex has never been a major part of their lives and motivation (and there are plenty of them). This pressure may be acute if you think you are about to lose the urge altogether, and can turn the peri-menopause into a classic mid-life crisis. You need to, borrowing a phrase from pop psychology, give yourself permission not to want sex. If you are in an active relationship, this is something you will need to discuss with your partner, and a time when the phrase "it's not you, it's me" will actually be true. Replacing oestrogen using HRT may well restore your libido, but it must be a decision based on your health and feelings. You need to be clear how important your sex life is before you make this the basis for embarking on HRT, and you should discuss all this with your partner if you have one.

Headaches

Believe it or not, there are more than 200 types of headaches, and a number of headache classification systems. The headaches that most of us experience are "primary" headaches, headaches that are not caused by any underlying disease or structural problems.

The majority of headaches can be classified as tension type headaches, or migraine headaches. The precise cause of head ache pain is not fully understood. The brain itself has no pain receptors, but the large blood vessels that supply the brain do, as do the cranial and spinal nerves, head and neck muscles, the membranes that surround the brain, and parts of the brainstem (the rear part of the brain that joins the spinal cord).

Migraine headache may consist of just a severe, usually throbbing or pounding, headache, but for many people there are other symptoms, such as visual disturbances, nausea and vomiting. True migraines can be severe and debilitating. There have been a number of theories about the cause of Migraine. For some time, it was believed that constriction, followed by sudden dilation of blood vessels in the brain, which activated pain receptors in the surrounding blood vessels. However, studies have failed to confirm this, and current theory is that chemicals released following activation of certain sensory nerves leads to inflammation of the membranes around the brain, and in some blood vessels. For sufferers, what is of more interest, is understanding what triggers a Migraine.

As well as certain food, atmospheric and emotional triggers, Migraine is often linked to hormone fluctuations, and many women associate them with the time just before a period when oestrogen levels drop. This is known as menstrual migraine. As you enter the Peri-menopause, hormone fluctuations become less predictable, as do the associated migraines, and you may experience them more often.

The good news is that, once your oestrogen levels settle as you enter the menopause proper, you may find that your migraines stop altogether, or, at least, become far less frequent, depending on what other factors trigger them for you.

Some types of HRT maintain a cyclical oestrogen pattern, and your migraines may continue, or you may even develop them even if you did not experience headaches as part of your natural cycle. Continuous HRT gives you stable oestrogen levels, and reduces the risk of Migraine. In fact, anything that stabilises your oestrogen levels can help to eliminate cyclical migraines.

Tension headaches are thought to be caused by activation of peripheral nerves in the head and neck muscles. The classic source of tension headaches is the sub-occipital muscle group at the base of the skull. This is a triangular group of muscles which supports the head, is involved in extension and rotation of the neck and head. You can feel them at the base of the skull. Try massaging them next time you have a headache.

Tension headaches are unlikely to be directly caused by the changes in your physiology at the menopause, or peri-menopause, but may be triggered by stress and anxiety that are directly associated with the menopause. Anything that helps to relieve stress and anxiety is likely to decrease the frequency of tension headaches (see chapter 3, Mood Swings).

Palpitations

Palpitations are irregular heartbeats. You may feel your heart speed up, or flutter, pound, or lose its rhythm. Palpitations do not usually last very long, a few minutes at worse.

Having your heart behave oddly can be quite alarming, but there is no reason to assume that you have a serious problem, particularly if they occur as you are going through the menopause.

Oestrogen affects the expansion and contraction of the coronary arteries, the large vessels that carry blood to the heart, and changes in oestrogen level, especially the erratic fluctuations that can occur as you pass into the menopause, can lead to changes in blood pressure and heart rhythm.

Oestrogen is also involved in the regulation of the autonomic nervous system, the system that controls the unconscious functions of the body (such as breathing and circulation), and, as a result, fluctuations in oestrogen level may also affect heart rate.

Changes in heart rhythm caused by menopausal hormone fluctuations, may be referred to as "non-threatening" arrhythmias – nevertheless, if you suddenly begin to experience palpitations, you should see your doctor to confirm that there is no other underlying cause.

What can you do about palpitations and arrhythmia?

HRT will prevent heart symptoms caused by low oestrogen, but there are other measures that can help to reduce the risk or the effect.

Like many symptoms or conditions, we experience, we can be made more vulnerable to palpitations and arrhythmias by lifestyle factors.

Avoid stimulants such as caffeine, alcohol and nicotine - a system that is artificially accelerated takes less to make it react abnormally.

Try and reduce your stress levels. Stress can lead to an increased heart rate, or just cause palpitations directly. The more you relax, the less intense the palpitations are likely to feel.

Build up your heart health with regular exercise and a healthy diet. A healthy diet will ensure that you maintain good levels of electrolytes such as potassium and magnesium, which are necessary for healthy heart function.

It has also been suggested that keeping well hydrated will reduce the strain on your heart and the likelihood of palpitations.

What can you do when palpitations happen?

First of all, try and relax. Breathe deeply, and remind yourself that, whatever you are feeling, there is nothing seriously wrong.

Coughing may help to reset your rhythm. You can also try holding your nose and closing your mouth while tensing your muscles as if trying to breathe out hard as if trying to blow up a balloon. This is thought to stimulate the vagus nerve which is heavily involved in heartbeat regulation. You can also try splashing your face with very cold water for the same reasons.

Bladder Problems

As we get older the risk of bladder incontinence increases.

The most common types of urinary incontinence in women are:

Stress incontinence, caused by weakened pelvic floor muscles. The most common symptoms are leakage of urine with coughing, laughing, sneezing, or lifting objects. Stress incontinence is common during perimenopause but typically doesn't worsen because of menopause.

Urge incontinence (also called "overactive bladder"), which is caused by overly active or irritated bladder muscles. The most common symptom is the frequent and sudden urge to urinate, with occasional leakage of urine.

The menopause is not necessarily the sole cause of loss of bladder control. The lining of the urethra, the tube that leads from the bladder to the exterior, is oestrogen sensitive, and becomes thinner and loses elasticity as oestrogen declines. However, obesity significantly increases the risk of incontinence, as it leads to pressure on the bladder. Pelvic floor muscles, weakened by earlier childbirth, and/or by age will decrease bladder control. Strengthening your pelvic floor muscles with exercise, and maintaining a healthy weight will reduce the risk of incontinence.

The use of oestrogen to treat bladder incontinence from the peri-menopause onwards remains controversial. However, the most consistent and promising results are with vaginal, rather than oral oestrogen preparations.

Some women experience an increase in urinary tract infections as they pass through the menopause. It is not always clear that the menopause is the direct cause. However, incontinence can be associated with an increased infection rate. The loss of oestrogen may also change the pH of the fluids in the vagina, making the environment more hospitable to hostile bacteria and increasing the risk of infection.

These are the twelve most frequently reported symptoms. It is not an exhaustive list. Some articles suggest that the menopause has as many as thirty-four symptoms, and it is true to say that the hormonal changes that lead to the menopause can have a broader spectrum of effects, including gum problems, brittle nails, hair loss, and a whole list of slightly alarming problems.

Don't panic. Very few women experience all of these symptoms. If we look back at the survey, 61 percent of women said that hot flushes had the greatest impact on their lives. This means that 39% of women felt that they did not. In fact, some women sail through the menopause, experiencing only the occasional symptom. At the other extreme, very few women find the menopause truly debilitating. Most of us sit somewhere in the middle. It does affect our lives, but we can manage it.

Legal Protection and Public Policy

If your symptoms are causing you problems at work, you need to be aware that, in the UK at least, the menopause is covered under the "Equality Act 2010". Cases have been won on the basis that symptoms may have a long term and substantial effect on day to day activities, bringing them within the definition of disability under section 6 of the Act.

Again, in the UK, the Civil Service has a working party that has published a toolkit to help employers support menopausal employees.

In the US and Australia there is increasing recognition of the need to understand and support employees suffering from significant menopausal symptoms.

Support notwithstanding, it is vital that you learn to control your menopause, and not let it control you.

In the following chapters we will look at what are, for most people, the most significant symptoms, and consider how they can be alleviated or controlled.

Chapter 2 - Hot Flushes and how to deal with them…

What is a Hot Flush?

Hot flushes are regarded by some medical practitioners and researchers as the only genuine symptoms of the menopause. Other symptoms are considered to be just a consequence of the ageing process. Whether this is true or not, there is no question that hot flushes are caused by the physiological changes associated with the menopause.

A typical description of a hot flush is a creeping feeling of intense warmth that quickly spreads across your whole body and face "right up to your brow". It typically lasts for several minutes. Others say the warmth is similar to the sensation of being under a sun bed, or feeling hot "like a furnace".

Some women experience a reddening and/or blotchiness of the face and neck which they find embarrassing. Others report what feels like a sudden rush of blood from their toes to the top of their head.

Some will sweat profusely as a result of the hot flush, and this can be the most uncomfortable and embarrassing aspect of all. Frequent, intense hot flushes, especially with sweating, can have a serious and debilitating impact on all aspects of life.

Are they inevitable?

Happily, not everyone suffers from hot flushes. In fact, 40% of women going through the menopause do not experience hot flushes at all. Of the remaining 60% that do, 70% will only have them for a year or less, 20- 25% for between a year and 5 years, and 5-10% for up to 10 years. The average duration is two years.

It should be said that these figures are based on women from Western Europe and North America. The incidence of hot flushes is lower in women of Asian origin, and the severity and duration are higher in women with African ancestry.

Frequency

Only 10 to 15% of women suffer badly enough to seek treatment, and this is usually because of the frequency as well as the intensity of flushes. Some women only experience a few flushes in a week. Others may have as many as 10 or more during the day and more at night. This is unusual, but when it does happen, and especially if these flushes are accompanied by sweating, you should seek help.

Why do they happen?

Hot flushes are known as the vasomotor symptom of the menopause. This simply means they relate to changes in the way blood vessels behave.

Like all mammals we are warm blooded. Our bodies have developed to maintain a constant temperature, whatever the surrounding environment. Everything is balanced to run at 37oC (98.4oF). In order to do this, we have a built in thermostat that detects when our internal temperature drifts. A significant change in our internal, or core temperature would have a disastrous effect on our physiology.

The hypothalamus, a small structure about the size of an almond, at the base of the brain, is responsible for detecting and acting on significant changes in body temperature.

If the hypothalamus senses that our body temperature is too high, it sends signals to the sweat glands in the skin, and to the capillaries, the small blood vessels that run under the surface of the skin. Sweating causes us to lose heat when the sweat evaporates, and the capillaries dilate so that a higher volume of blood passes just below the surface of the skin causing us to lose more heat. This increased blood flow is responsible for the flushing, or reddening of the skin that occurs when we are hot.

If our body temperature becomes too low, the hypothalamus sends out signals to our muscles which cause us to shiver.

There is a narrow temperature within which the body tolerates changes without triggering a reaction. Research suggests that during the menopause, some of us will see this range reduced, so that the slightest temperature fluctuation will trigger a response. If the temperature so much as flickers upwards, we will experience a hot flush as the body attempts to cool itself.

Inevitably the underlying cause is the reduction in oestrogen. Oestrogen is involved in the regulation of temperature and a decline in oestrogen results in the narrowing of our range of temperature tolerance. In other words, our sensitivity to temperature changes goes up as our oestrogen levels fall. While the precise mechanism is not entirely clear, there is plenty of evidence that putting oestrogen back into the system (via HRT) restores temperature tolerance to normal.

However, there are a number of other hormones and neurotransmitters involved in temperature regulation, and over time the body adapts to the lack of oestrogen, and the hot flushes stop.

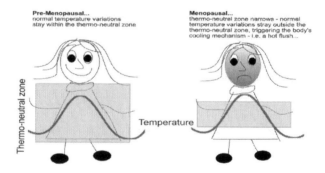

What can we do about Hot Flushes?

Lifestyle

Before we resort to medication there are a number of lifestyle changes or adjustments to consider. The obvious one is to avoid any activity that is likely to raise our core temperature - saunas, hot baths, for example.

Try and keep room temperatures slightly cool, especially at night. Even without hot flushes to worry about, we sleep better if our body temperature is slightly lowered.

Wear natural fibres. These allow moisture from the body to evaporate, and keep skin temperature lower than man-made fibres.

Make sure you get plenty of exercise. This may seem counter intuitive, as exercise itself is likely to make you hot. However, regular exercise increases the efficiency of your vasomotor systems - the systems that control your blood vessels. It also reduces stress and stress hormones, such as serotonin, are also involved in the initiation of hot flushes.

Exercise, as well as a healthy diet will help you to keep your weight in check. If you are overweight, you will have a more difficult time dealing with hot flushes. Your body will struggle with temperature control as it has more insulation than our metabolism is designed to cope with, and cooling will be harder and take longer.

Food and Drink

You should avoid caffeine and alcohol if you suffer badly from hot flushes. Both raise your core temperature directly or indirectly.

Spicy food, specifically food containing chillies, or chilli products, is thought to be a major trigger for hot flushes. There are no major studies to support this, but none to contradict it either. If you are a lover of chillies you might want to do your own experiment.

Spikes in blood sugar levels can trigger a stress reaction which, in turn, may trigger a hot flush. Reducing your sugar intake may also reduce your hot flushes.

A generally healthy diet, along with a generally healthy lifestyle may not stop your hot flushes, but it will help you to deal with them. If you feel well, relaxed and positive, you are less likely to dwell on them, and more likely to cope.

It has been suggested that eating a diet rich in soy will help to reduce hot flushes, particularly as in countries where soy is a traditional part of the diet fewer women have hot flushes, and those who do, have fewer than the average woman in Western Europe or the USA. However, the evidence (see appendix 1.) does not support this theory. Trials have shown that increasing the amount of soy in the diet has no effect on the frequency or duration of hot flushes, so there has to be some other explanation as to why women in the far east have fewer problems with temperature control during the menopause.

Supplements

A number of herbal supplements such as Black Cohosh are marketed on the basis that they will relieve hot flushes and other menopausal symptoms. There are no scientific trials that support this, and Black Cohosh has a number of unpleasant and potentially serious side effects - the problems with this, and plant oestrogens in general are covered elsewhere in this book (see page 27).

No multi-mineral/vitamin combination will stop your hot flushes, even if they have a trade name that suggest they are designed to relieve menopausal symptoms. The manufacturers are simply trying to exploit your discomfort.

The only vitamin shown to have any effect is folic acid. One study has shown a daily 5mg dose of folic acid is more effective than placebo in reducing flushes. If you want to try this, you could take a supplement, or you could increase the amount of green vegetables, pulses, bread and pasta in your diet. All of these are good sources of folic acid.

Alternative Therapies

Acupuncture has been proposed as a way of relieving hot flushes, as has Yoga. Sadly, there is no evidence that these will have any direct effect, although relaxation and slow breathing exercises may help to reduce the intensity of hot flushes.

Cognitive behavioural therapy (CBT – see Appendix 2) has also been proposed as a way of reducing hot flushes, and is recommended by the American Menopause Society. In the UK the National Institute for Clinical Excellence recommends it for relieving anxiety related to the menopause, but not for hot flushes.

Magnets, Bracelets and other Paraphernalia

If you google "hot flushes", as well as the vitamins, and herbal remedies, you may come across the suggestion that buying a (very expensive) magnet and putting it in your underwear will help with hot flushes. While it is always best to keep an open mind where any form of medicine is concerned, there is no possible mechanism by which a magnet in your underwear can affect hot flushes or other menopausal symptoms. The same goes for wearing bracelets, magnetic, silver copper, or any material. Neither will healing stones or crystals affect the response of your hypothalamus to changes in core temperature.

It is infinitely possible that you will speak to someone who swears their hot flushes reduced when they wore their magnet/bracelet/crystal, and they will certainly be telling you the truth. However, this is likely to occur at some time, and it is likely that the use of the device merely coincided with the point at which the hot flushes subside. Those who bought them and failed to experience any effect are not very likely to shout about it (see appendix 1 Evidence).

There is also underwear advertised that is designed to help with hot flushes. Other than soaking up the sweat, it is difficult to understand how a vest can make things better. However, the marketing material suggests that these vests are nothing short of a miracle. You need to make up your own mind about this.

Medication

If you really cannot live with your hair trigger thermostat, you may need to resort to prescription medication. There are a number of prescription drugs that will give you some relief.

HRT

Replacing oestrogen using HRT will work for most people (see chapter 4). However, some women cannot use HRT for medical reasons, and others prefer not to as they are concerned about the risks and side effects. There are, however, a number of other drugs that have been found to be effective.

Antidepressants

The family of antidepressants known as selective serotonin re-uptake inhibitors (SSRIs), and selective norepinephrine re-uptake inhibitors have both been shown to reduce the incidence and severity of hot flushes. Serotonin and Norepinephrine are neurotransmitters that are involved in temperature regulation so it ought not to be a surprise that something that affects the levels of these chemicals would have an impact on hot flushes. The effect of these drugs was an accidental discovery. A number of studies have now been conducted that suggest that hot flushes may be reduced by up to 65%. The most common side effect of these drugs are dry mouth, nausea, constipation, and sleep disruption, although most of these usually resolve after a week or two. For women who are not prepared to take HRT, or live with their hot flushes, this discomfort may be worth putting up with for a short time.

Clonidine

Clonidine is a drug used to control blood pressure. It reduces blood pressure in the brain by causing some blood vessels to dilate, to open up, and this seems to reduce the frequency and intensity of hot flushes for some women.

The side effects are dizziness, nausea, constipation and dry mouth. As with the antidepressants, these symptoms usually disappear within a short time.

Gabapentin

Gabapentin is used to treat epilepsy, and belongs to a family of drugs known as anticonvulsants, that prevent seizures. It is also used to treat nerve pain, particularly that caused by shingles, phantom pain in amputees, and in the prevention of migraine. The mechanism by which it reduces hot flushes is not clear, but some studies have shown to be as effective as the SSRI antidepressants and even oestrogen. Side effects include dizziness, drowsiness and tiredness, nausea and vomiting, and lack of coordination. These should pass as the body adjusts.

If some of these drugs seem a little extreme, it is worth bearing in mind that, for a small minority of women, hot flushes are extremely debilitating. If this is you, then you should not be afraid to try drug treatment. Your doctor will not prescribe them unless they are safe for you to take. If the side effects are transient but your hot flushes are not, then the trade off in discomfort may be worth it.

New Developments

A new drug, MLE4901, is in the process of development which directly block the action of one of the chemicals involved in the mechanism that causes hot flushes. It has been highly successful in trials and appears to have no significant side effects. We will have to wait a while for this to be available, but it is encouraging that there is active research, and that these symptoms are taken seriously by the medical profession and the pharmaceutical industry.

Where do we go from here?

For many of us hot flushes are the most significant, uncomfortable, and even miserable aspect of the menopause. If this is you, and you are prepared to take medication, you should discuss your experience with your family doctor to decide what would be best and safest for you.

Otherwise, the best approach would be to keep your stress levels as low as possible, learn some slow breathing techniques, lose some weight (if you need to), and eat a healthy diet.

Taking exercise, and lowering your stress levels may not stop your hot flushes - but you will be in a better mental and physical state to cope with them.

Chapter 3 - Mood Swings and how to deal with them

What is a Mood?

A mood, according to the Oxford English Dictionary, is a temporary state of mind or feeling. It is a transient frame of mind that influences the way we see the world. Something causes us to feel happiness, sadness, anger or some other emotion, in a way that is separate from our underlying state of mind. If you wake up feeling good because you have slept well, and you have positive plans for the day, you may find you feelings changing suddenly, but temporarily when you stub your toe in the shower, or find you are out of toothpaste. This "bad mood" will probably pass with the pain, or when you find a new tube of toothpaste. Your underlying state of mind will eventually assert itself.

On the other hand, you may be feeling sad or stressed because of events in your life, and hearing a favourite, or uplifting piece of music, or a friendly voice on the phone can cheer you up for a while. It has not changed anything materially, but somehow it has put you in a better "mood".

How does this work?

The brain interprets events and governs our responses. An event might be external - the sun has come out and the light and warmth make us feel cheerful - or internal - a pain or some other chemical event. When the brain detects an event, it will alter our physiology in the most advantageous way - at least that is how it is supposed to work.

Buried deep in the brain is the limbic system. It is thought to be one of the oldest and most primitive parts of the brain, and is made up of a number of structures, including the hippocampus, the amygdala, and the hypothalamus, all of which are involved in emotions in some way. These types of structures are found in the brain of many other species. What we think of as moods and emotions represent our response to our environment. These reactions come about by a combination of input from our senses, memories, and neurotransmitters, the chemical messengers of the nervous system, which convey messages to the limbic system and from the limbic system to the rest of the brain and the body.

Waking up on that sunny day, sends messages from the eyes, via the visual cortex, the part of the brain that processes images, which trigger a memory which tells us that conditions are good for hunting or gathering, or, in a more modern setting, for going to the beach, doing the gardening, or just for feeling the warmth of the sun (which impacts positively on another part of our brain and physiology...but this is another story). The fact is, the brain, via our memories, makes positive associations, and sends out messages using neurotransmitters

transmitters, that make us feel energised and positive, the right frame of mind for getting on with tasks.

On the other hand, there are sudden events that trigger memories that say we must act quickly and immediately, things we recognise as urgent or dangerous. In this case the brain will send out an entirely different combination of neurotransmitters, setting up a fight or flight response, raising your heartbeat, diverting blood to the muscles, and generally setting you up for drastic action.

These systems operate regardless of the source of the stimulus. Watching a sad film gives us feelings of sadness, despite the fact that nothing has actually happened to us. We react to what we see, hear and feel, usually before we have a chance to rationalise it.

Fortunately, unlike other species, we have brain centres that are involved in longer term planning, and prevent us from acting entirely on the messages from the limbic system. As a result, we do not beat the person who pushes in front of us in the supermarket queue over the head with our umbrella, or a handy baguette, because they are getting between us and our source of food. Higher brain centres exercise restraint, based on our knowledge of the possible consequences if we give way to an impulse for violence.

Not all of our moods have an external source. Having understood that the brain regulates our moods, it is also important to understand that the brain may also create them.

Anyone who has experienced a spontaneous panic attack will tell you that their feelings are as intense as if they were genuinely under threat, whereas, in reality this was just a change in their brain chemistry.

What causes changes in Brain Chemistry?

Outside of real events there are factors that affect our physiology and brain chemistry resulting in mood changes. Sleep is vital for maintenance of our systems. Insufficient sleep alters brain chemistry, often leading to a feeling of "low" mood, or an increased susceptibility to feelings of anger or irritability. In other words, not only can changes in chemistry induce mood changes, but they may lower our trigger threshold for certain types of moods.

Low blood sugar may also produce feelings of irritability and anxiety.

…And then there are the mood changes we associate with different hormonal states.

The Menopause and Mood Swings

Peri-menopausal and menopausal women often describe sudden feelings of anxiety, or of being "overwhelmed", or of feeling tearful for no reason. Others report feelings of depression, and some experience rage, again, for no obvious reason.

Oestrogen is linked with the production of serotonin, one of the neurotransmitters involved in the regulation of emotions and moods.

Low serotonin is associated with low mood and confusion, high serotonin with happiness, and an increased ability to learn and carry out complex tasks. In the middle is calm. Very high serotonin levels result in a state similar to sedation, and very low is associated with some debilitating psychiatric conditions. Clearly, regulation of serotonin is essential for our emotional health, and most types of medication used in the treatment of depression have the effect of maintaining levels of serotonin in the blood.

Oestrogen slows down the rate at which serotonin is taken out of the blood stream, and also increases the sensitivity of the brain to serotonin by increasing the number of serotonin receptors on the brain cells.

During the "perimenopause" the levels of oestrogen may rise sharply and then drop.

When oestrogen rises so do our serotonin levels. When it crashes, our serotonin levels do the same. Most of us are familiar with the effects of these types of changes as they are responsible for the emotional changes many of us experience just before a period, as oestrogen levels drop dramatically (albeit temporarily).

So throughout the perimenopausal and menopausal stage we may be experiencing the equivalent of random PMT.

Serotonin is not the only neurotransmitter involved in oestrogen related mood swings. Oestrogen also slows down that rate at which both dopamine and norepinephrine are absorbed. Low oestrogen results in low levels of these neurotransmitters. Dopamine is involved in regulating mood, and our feelings of reward and pleasure. Low levels lead to depressive moods. On the other hand, very high levels of dopamine lead to feelings of aggression, irritability, impulsivity, and ultimately psychosis. High levels of oestrogen may keep dopamine levels too high. This explains the feelings of anger and aggression that some women experience as part of PMT - oestrogen levels are at their highest just before they plummet at the end of a cycle.

Norepinephrine regulates the fight and flight response to threat, as well as alertness and energy, and at high levels produces feelings of stress and anxiety. Break it down too fast and we are left without energy and the capacity to respond to stressful situations. If levels build up, we may be overcome with anxiety. Oestrogen regulates the levels of norepinephrine through the same mechanism as dopamine.

As a result, during the peri-menopause, the impact of changing oestrogen levels on serotonin, dopamine and norepinephrine can result in moods that fluctuate from depression to rage.

This is, of course the extreme. Many of us will survive with occasional feelings of anxiety or depression, and some will barely notice a difference.

What can we do about Mood Swings?

Exercise

Exercise is a great mood enhancer. Not only does it release endorphins, another group of neurotransmitters that give us a natural "high", but it also raises the levels of dopamine, norepinephrine and serotonin. If your dipping oestrogen levels are getting you down, exercise can help to redress the balance. Any form of exercise, a vigorous walk, or even climbing a flight of stairs, can help.

It may be the last thing you feel like doing when you are in a low mood, but it is the quickest way to correct your rebellious physiology. Most of us would not hesitate to take a pill, side effects and all, if it was going to make us feel better instantly. Exercise can do exactly that, and the side effects are all good.

If your mood has swung into an angry phase, the increased levels of serotonin brought about by exercise can calm you, and you can burn off the surplus energy of outrage.

Some people find it easier to take exercise in an organised form. You do not necessarily have to join a class. There are plenty of online courses, and You Tube is a great source of self-help videos. On the other hand, joining a class and getting involved may be exactly what you need - we are all different.

Diet

Eat a healthy diet. Go easy on caffeine, sugar and alcohol, all of which may have effects both directly on mood, and indirectly on the important mood regulating neurotransmitters.

Eating a healthy diet, low in processed foods, artificial colourings, salt and sugar, can improve your energy levels and your general state of health, which will put you in a better state to deal with mood swings.

Diet is also important in helping to control or reduce your weight. How does this help with mood? Low self - esteem has a tendency to creep in with the menopause, as a manifestation of low mood, but also as a symptom of our concerns about ageing. Staving off middle-age spread, or shedding surplus pounds can help with this. As you lose weight, exercise, with all its mood enhancing benefits, becomes easier.

Go for

- Complex carbohydrates. Whole grain breads, and cereals help raise serotonin levels and can reduce depression.

- Omega-3 Fatty acids. Salmon, tuna, walnuts, almonds, and flaxseeds are all rich in this essential fatty acid.

- Protein. Nuts, chicken, cheese, eggs, are all good sources of protein.

Avoid

- Processed and red meats. Limit consumption of processed and red meats because they contain high amounts of saturated fats and decrease the body's ability to metabolize estrogen.

- Sugars. Eating excessive amounts of sugar can impair the immune system and limit the liver's ability to metabolize estrogen.

- Caffeine. Avoid caffeine entirely or consume in moderation.

- Fast Food. Trans fat can clog arteries and consumption can also lead to weight gain and hormone imbalance.

Medication

HRT

By restoring your hormone balance, HRT may eliminate mood swings. It is important that you find the right preparation and dose. Getting this wrong may alter the moods you are experiencing but not eliminate the swings from one state to another (see chapter 4).

Anti-depressants

Particular types of anti-depressants including Prozac, may help with other symptoms of the menopause, but are not a great idea when it comes to mood swings. Nor are any type of tranquillisers.

Depression is a chronic state (see below). Mood swings, by definition, mean that your emotions are far from constant.

Unfortunately, there is no form in which you can take in serotonin directly by mouth, as serotonin cannot cross from the blood stream directly into the brain. However, you can take 5 hydroxytryptophan, or 5 HTP. Our bodies convert 5-HTP into serotonin, and there is some evidence that taking 5 HTP by mouth does raise serotonin levels, and can therefore help to control mood swings.

Dietary Supplements/Herbal Remedies

There are a number of supplements that are claimed to help with mood swings, but most of these are considered to have some impact on all menopausal symptoms. St John's Wort may have some impact on hot flushes, but the real evidence for its effectiveness relates to depression. It may work as a mood enhancer, as well as a straightforward relief for depression, but it must be taken for some time before the effects can be felt, and it interferes with a number of other medications, so it is important that you consult your doctor before trying it.

Ginseng is one of the most popular medicinal herbs. There a number of different types, with slightly differing components, which make studies on effectiveness confusing. However, a meta-analysis, which is an analysis of all the properly controlled clinical trials that have been published, failed to demonstrate any impact on menopausal mood swings. Some of the trials suggested that there might be an impact, but these were considered to be biased. The problem with many clinical trials lies in the fact that those who conduct them have a vested interest in finding a positive outcome. This is sometimes obvious in the way they are conducted and the way in which the results are analysed. In the same way we are more likely to accept something we want to believe, those with an interest are more likely to publish the results that work best for them. In the end, if you have used ginseng, and believe in its effects, you may also find that it helps with your mood swings - otherwise, there is no reason for you to try it, especially as it does clash with some anti-depressant prescription drugs. You should also check with your doctor before taking ginseng if you are taking any medication to prevent blood clots.

Kava kava, a traditional remedy from the South Pacific, used to be recommended for anxiety associated with the menopause, and was shown to have some effect, but has been banned, at least in the UK, as it was shown to cause liver damage.

Plant (phyto) Oestrogens

There are a number of compounds found in plants that are chemically similar to oestrogen. It would be wonderful if, instead of taking HRT in the form of a prescribed pill we could eat the right selection of vegetables and get the same effect. The problem is that, while these compounds are similar to oestrogen, they are not exactly the same.

Black cohosh is one of the most popular supplements taken by women with peri-menopausal and menopausal symptoms. Black cohosh is a perennial herb of the buttercup family from North America, also known as bugbane, rattleweed, and black snakeroot (not particularly promising names...). Native Americans began using it centuries ago for the treatment of menstrual irregularities, menopause symptoms, and to ease childbirth. There is no conclusive evidence of its effectiveness in reducing oestrogen related mood swings. There are, however, concerns about possible side effects, including liver damage. The North American Menopause Society has stopped recommending Black Cohosh, as there is a long list of other possible side effects, including, like ginseng, problems for those on medication such as warfarin, for preventing blood clots.

Soy is a major source of phytoestrogens. It is also a more widespread dietary component than most people suspect, being present in up to 60% of processed foods. Again there is no conclusive evidence for a positive therapeutic effect in women suffering from peri-menopausal mood swings.

These compounds are referred to as endocrine disruptors, because they will interfere in some way with hormone processes and pathways. Man-made endocrine disruptors with similar structures include DDT - not something you would imagine taking for your mood swings, and phthalates, substances used in the manufacture of plastics, known to cause problems in the environment by disrupting the reproductive function of fish if leached into seas and waterways.

The term oestrogen refers to a number of related chemicals. The body itself makes several different forms. HRT uses very specifically structured, targeted compounds based on the precise natural form of oestrogen that we require to maintain our emotional equilibrium among other things. While phytoestrogens are from the same chemical family, the resemblance is just not close enough.

Alternative Therapies

Acupuncture

The evidence for acupuncture as a way of relieving mood swings in the peri-menopausal is confusing. Acupuncture practitioners, organisations and support groups, and fans of acupuncture in general, clearly believe that it is effective in relieving peri-menopausal and menopausal symptoms. However, there seems to be no independent medical evidence to show a clear connection between acupuncture and relief of mood swings. An information leaflet published by the Royal College of Obstetricians and Gynaecologists lists acupuncture as being safe but ineffective against peri-menopausal mood swings.

If you have used acupuncture and found it useful in helping you to relax, or to fight depression, you may find that it helps with mood swings. In other words, if you believe in it, it may work for you. Otherwise there simply is no real clinical evidence one way or the other, so you will need to make up your own mind whether it is something you would like to try.

The same goes for reflexology, reiki, and all other complementary therapies. If you already have experience of these and they have had a positive effect for other conditions you may wish to try them, but bear in mind there is no scientific evidence to suggest that they will help with peri-menopausal mood swings.

So you really don't want to take HRT…

Aside from HRT, the best remedies for peri-menopausal mood swings, based on the existing evidence are:

Healthy diet and weight loss

Exercise

St John's Wort (if you really need to take something).

Finding a distraction

The worst thing you can do is to dwell on the fact that you are experiencing low moods more often during this phase in your life. It is a phase and it will pass. Try and remember this. It is your chemistry misbehaving, not your life going off the rails.

Set yourself some goals to lose weight or to exercise more often - anything that will give you a sense of achievement.

Take up an absorbing hobby or craft, something that is a distraction and gives you a different focus, and can give you a sense of achievement. Again, you might be happier doing this alone, or joining a group or class might help by giving you a change of environment and different company.

If this all seems too simple, and you are feeling overwhelmed by misery to the extent that you struggle to get out of bed, or to motivate yourself even to help yourself, try and remember that this a chemical imbalance. It is not life throwing you a worse hand than ever. Try and see your feelings in the same way you might deal with a physical pain. It hurts, and it is tough, but it will pass, and faster if you do make an effort. It is a process that you need to go through. If your low mood persists over more than a day or so, then you may be experiencing something more serious than mood swings (see depression below).

Depression - the D word..

The menopause does not cause depression. Being peri-menopausal does not cause depression. Unpredictable bouts of low mood are not the same as depression which is a chronic (ongoing) condition. The fact that you may be prescribed anti-depressants to combat mood swings does not mean you are necessarily clinically depressed. Depression is an illness - the menopause is not.

Nevertheless, women in mid-life do suffer from depression, and this is often to do with other changes in our lives, such as children leaving home, or even simply coming to terms with the fact that we are getting older.

Fear of ageing is a little irrational when you consider the alternative, but for some women, the fact that they will no longer be able to get pregnant (whether they wanted to or not), but especially if they have not completed their family, is distressing, and can lead to feelings of depression.

For some women the menopause represents the crossing of a bridge from youth into old age. They imagine that, once their periods stop, they will rapidly collapse into a wrinkled unattractive heap, and this is, understandably, a depressing notion, even if it is utterly untrue. If your happiness depends on the way you are perceived by others, and your feeling of self-worth is based on how attractive you consider yourself to be, or how you perform in life relative to the expectations of others, and not on how you feel about yourself and your achievements, you will be far more vulnerable to negative feelings, moods and ultimately, depression.

Some women use the term depression for their mood swings because they think it will be easier for other people to understand. This, however, carries with it the danger of becoming a self-fulfilling prophecy. Say that you are depressed often enough and you may come to believe it.

Take a positive view of the changes you are going through. Make plans for the future and keep yourself fit and occupied in the present. And stay away from the D word...

Chapter 4 - Hormone Replacement Therapy

What is HRT?

Hormone replacement therapy is exactly that. We take, usually in the form of pills or patches, carefully measured doses of the oestrogen, the disappearance of which causes us so much discomfort.

Putting back oestrogen does not restore our reproductive function. Our ovaries are exhausted. There are no eggs left to ovulate. What HRT does is address the other effects, such as temperature regulation (hot flushes), changes in the brain (depression, mood swings), energy levels (fatigue and that horrible flu-like aching).

Starting HRT can relieve symptoms in a matter of weeks, sometimes even in a few days. Many women find they feel better on HRT than they have in a long time. Some effects of oestrogen depletion in the peri-menopause are subtle and you may not notice them until they are gone.

It all sounds rather miraculous - a veritable magic bullet. For some of us it really does work this well and fast. So why is there so much controversy about HRT?

Firstly, it just does not work that well for everyone. Some women struggle to find the right dose or the right preparation, and some simply cannot tolerate exogenous (from the outside, not produced by the body) hormones.

Some women may be advised against HRT for health reasons, particularly those who are struggling with high blood pressure - and there are the well publicised risks.

It is important to have accurate information about the risks, the benefits, the types of HRT, and what would be best for you before you make up your mind.

The Benefits of HRT

By stabilizing oestrogen levels HRT can:

Significantly reduce, and in many cases, eliminate hot flushes, within four weeks of starting treatment.

- Alleviates both low mood and mood swings caused by fluctuating oestrogen

- Relieve vaginal dryness and improve sexual function

- Protects against osteoporosis and significantly reduces the risk of fractures. The protection continues for some years after stopping HRT

- Help to maintain muscle mass and skin elasticity, and may also help with wound healing.

- Helps to restore sleep patterns, and relieve muscle aches and pains

- There is evidence that HRT reduces the risk of heart disease if it is started soon after the onset of the menopause. Research also suggests that the risks of Alzheimer's, and other forms of dementia, are reduced by long term use of HRT, but the evidence is not strong. The risk of colo-rectal and stomach cancer may also be reduced by the long term use of HRT, but further trials are needed to confirm this.

So what are the Risks?

The risks of HRT have been well publicised. Naturally you need to be aware of them, but it is vital that your decision making is based on accurate information and not newspaper headlines (see statistics below).

You also need to bear in mind that lifestyle factors such as lack of exercise, poor diet, obesity, smoking and alcohol are likely to have a greater impact than HRT on your chances of developing conditions such as stroke, heart disease and cancer.

Stroke

There is evidence that women over 60 taking HRT by mouth have an increased risk of stroke and thrombosis, leading to an additional 6 to 8 cases per thousand (according to a 2015 study). 8 cases per thousand is actually 0.8 percent, so the risk increases by less than 1 percent.

Another recent study suggests that using patches instead of pills eliminates this increase in risk.

Cancer

HRT is also associated with an increased risk of both ovarian and breast cancer. On the face of it this is enough to put anyone off taking it. This is where we have to take a serious look at the statistics.

Breast Cancer

In women aged between 50 and 79 who are not taking HRT there are, on average, 9 to 17 cases of breast cancer in every 1000. This equates to a risk of 0.9 to 1.7%. In women in the same age group who are taking HRT, there are likely to be 13 to 23 cases, around six more in every thousand, an increase of 0.6%. The risk is higher for women taking combined oestrogen/progestogen HRT, and highest in those who have been taking it for more than 10 years.

A family history of breast cancer will increase your personal risk, and women with a family history of breast cancer may be advised against taking HRT.

Ovarian Cancer

Ovarian cancer is much rarer. In women taking HRT the risk increases from 2 cases in 2000 to 3 cases in 2000, an increase of 0.05%. The five-year survival rate for ovarian cancer is 46% compared to 87% for breast cancer, but the chances of developing it are much lower, and the impact of HRT is also much smaller.

Endometrial Cancer

Endometrial cancer, also referred to as womb or uterine cancer, occurs as a result of overgrowth of the lining of the womb.

Cancer relating to the womb is the fourth most common type of cancer in females, and represents 5% of all cancer cases in women. 28 new cases per 100,000 women will be diagnosed each year, according to Cancer Research UK.

However, the highest risk factor for uterine cancer is obesity. 34% of cases are related to obesity, while only 1% are related to the use of HRT, and then the risk is lower if you are using a combined oestrogen-progestogen preparation.

Maintaining a healthy weight will have a far more significant effect on your risk of endometrial cancer than stopping HRT.

The 5-year survival rate for uterine cancer is 79%

Should I take HRT?

You are only likely to consider HRT if you are finding your menopausal symptoms difficult to live with. The truth is that HRT is the only therapy that is likely to give you real relief. For the vast majority of woman who take it, that relief is significant, if not complete - and the vast majority of women who take it do not suffer significant health problems as a result of taking HRT.

You will need to do your own risk/benefit analysis. If you do decide to take it, remember you can change your preparation or stop if either it doesn't not work for you, or you feel that you could cope without it.

if you decide you would like to try HRT, make sure your doctor listens to your needs and your wishes. Some doctors are enthusiastic about HRT (especially female doctors who are taking it), while others are reluctant to prescribe. You need to talk to a doctor or nurse who will be objective, so that you get the right advice, and the right support. After all, this is your decision, about your life and your health.

How do I take HRT?

There are two main factors that will determine the type of HRT you should take:-

- How far into the menopause are you?

- Have you had a hysterectomy?

If you have had a hysterectomy you only need to take oestrogen. You can take this as a daily pill or a weekly or twice weekly patch.

If you still have your womb you will need a regime that includes progestogen (an artificial form of progesterone) as well as oestrogen.

Before the menopause, oestrogen causes the lining of the womb to thicken, but the growth of the lining or endometrium, is limited by the progesterone that is produced in the second half of the cycle, and the lining will then be shed once a month during your period. Taking oestrogen as part of HRT will have the same effect, but as you are no longer producing progesterone, or having periods, you will need to take some progesterone (usually in the form of the artificial progestogen). Taking oestrogen alone will lead to an overgrowth of the womb lining, and a risk of cancer, but adding progesterone to your HRT significantly reduces this risk.

Cyclical or continuous HRT

If you are still having periods, or have only just stopped, you should be prescribed a cyclical form of HRT. This involves taking a daily pill, but for those of us who were used to taking the contraceptive pill, this is a familiar routine.

Monthly Cyclical HRT

This is the most common form of cyclical HRT. Your tablet will be divided into packs of 28 pills. For the first 14 days you take pills containing only oestrogen. For the second half of the cycle the pills contain oestrogen and progestogen. At the end of each cycle you will have a bleed, very much like a normal period.

3 Monthly Cyclical HRT

If you are having very irregular periods, or have just stopped, you may be offered three monthly cyclical HRT, which involves taking oestrogen every day, and progestogen for 14 days every 13 weeks, giving you a bleed every three months. This may seem more convenient but involves less progestogen, which means you are less well protected against endometrial cancer, so you may prefer to opt for the monthly regime.

Continuous HRT

If your periods have stopped, you may be prescribed a continuous form of HRT. Each tablet contains both oestrogen, and progestogen, and you will not have a monthly bleed. Understandably, many women find this more convenient.

HRT Patches

You can also have continuous HRT in the form of skin patches. These patches are impregnated with oestrogen and progestogen which are absorbed through the skin into the blood stream. In terms of benefits, there is very little difference between tablets and patches. However, there is an advantage to the patches if you have a history of liver problems as the hormones are absorbed directly, and do not pass through the liver, as with hormones taken by mouth.

Intra-uterine System (IUS)

This involves a small T shaped device, similar to the contraceptive coil (IUD), that can only be inserted or removed by a doctor or nurse. Once in the womb it releases progestogen which acts directly on the lining of the womb to keep it thin and reduce the risk of cancer from overgrowth of the womb lining or endometrium. The effects may last for up to four years before it will need to be removed or replaced.

The National institute of clinical excellence in the UK, recommends the use of a coil, with oestrogen delivered via transdermal (through the skin) patches, as the least risky form of HRT, with the highest level of protection against endometrial cancer. However, some women struggle with the idea of having a coil fitted, and find combined pills or patches much easier to deal with.

HRT Gel

Oestrogen gel may be used in tandem with a coil, or progestogen tablets. It should be rubbed on the skin daily.

Vaginal Oestrogen

If the only problem you are worried about is vaginal dryness, you can use a vaginal cream or gel containing oestrogen, or pessaries that are inserted in the vagina and release oestrogen over time. There are virtually no risks associated with what is known as "local" (I.e. In the area where the problem occurs) application of oestrogen, so if your other menopausal symptoms are mild enough to cope with, then this may be the answer for you.

Implants

Implants are the least common way of taking HRT. They are more often used by women who have had their ovaries and womb removed and have become menopausal prematurely as a result. They may require HRT over a very long period of time, and an implant is more convenient and reliable. A small incision under local anaesthetic, and a pellet containing oestrogen is placed in the fatty tissue that lies just under the skin. The wound is closed with a stitch. As the implant wears out, menopausal symptoms will start to return. This can happen any time from 6 to 9 months after the implant is put in place.

Some doctors recommend that implants are not used after the age of 50, around the time that the menopause would have occurred naturally. After this age implants are considered to carry higher risks than the other forms of HRT.

The use and availability of implants has declined in recent years. In the UK Oestradiol implants are no longer licensed. However, this does not mean they are not available. Some clinics will prescribe and treat women who have undergone a natural menopause with oestrogen implants. If you are offered an implant you will also need to take progesterone, as a pill or a patch.

Bioidentical HRT

The hormones contained in conventional HRT preparations are often from animal sources and may not be identical in molecular terms to those that humans produce. Bio identical HRT contains hormones derived from plant sources and are manufactured to be identical in structure to the human forms. Some of these are present in commonly prescribed forms of HRT, but there is a market in "tailor made" bioidenticals, which have a formulation apparently based on the hormone levels present in your saliva. For some reason, hormones from plant sources are considered to be more "natural" than those derived from animals, and the idea of a personalized preparation apparently has some appeal. Many of these preparations are not approved by drug licensing bodies (e.g. the MHRA in the UK, and the FDA in the USA), and there is no evidence that fine tuning your dosage based on saliva makes any difference. It will however, cost you a great deal more. If you are worried about taking conventional HRT because of perceived risks of, for example, breast cancer, remember these risks are associated with taking oestrogen, and bioidentical HRT is still oestrogen, even if it has a pretty flower on the packet and costs you more. The best approach, as always, is to look carefully at the evidence of both risks and benefits, before you make a decision as to what to take, and as ever, be on the lookout for the unscrupulous practitioners who aim to take advantage of anyone desperate for a remedy.

Practicalities

Blood pressure checks

With all HRT you will need regular blood pressure checks, and you should report anything unusual to your doctor as soon as possible.

Oral HRT

If you are taking HRT in the form of tablets, you should aim to take them at the same time each day. There is no prescribed "best" time to take your HRT. Many women find it easier to take them at night as part of a bed time routine, especially those who were used to taking the contraceptive pill. Others find that taking HRT at night causes problems sleeping, and prefer to take their tablets in the morning. You should experiment to find out what works best for you.

If you miss a tablet, and you notice less than 12 hours after you should have taken it, you should take it immediately. If it is more than 12 hours since you should have taken it, you will need to miss that dose. Missing a single dose will not do you any harm.

Patches

HRT patches should be stuck on the lower part of your stomach, or on your buttock. Make sure your clothing is not likely to rub it off. You can bathe or shower as normal, and swimming is not a problem.

If a patch does come off, put on a new one, but change this at the time you would have changed the original.

Never put a patch in exactly the same place as the last one. Allow a couple of weeks before putting a patch in a place you have previously used.

Oestrogen Gel

Oestrogen gel should be rubbed on the skin every day. It can be applied to any convenient skin surface, but the breasts should be avoided. If you have not had a hysterectomy you will need to add progestogen in the form of tablets, or via a coil.

Mirena Coil

There may be some pain when the coil is inserted, and you may have some cramps. There are small risks of infection and of the device being expelled. You will be shown how to feel for the two threads that hang down into the vagina that tell you the coil is still in place. If you feel that the device has moved, or you can no longer feel the threads, you should check with your doctor immediately.

HRT Side Effects

As with most medication HRT has some side effects. Not everyone will suffer, and in any case it is worth persevering as these will usually pass in a few weeks.

The most common side effects (affecting more than 1 in 10) with combined HRT are headache, breast pain and breast tenderness.

The next set of side effects (affecting up to 1 in 10) include mood changes, changes in sex drive and difficulty sleeping. There are a good few more, but, like these, many of the side effects on this list are difficult to distinguish from the symptoms of the menopause that we are trying to relieve.

Do not let these put you off. You will only be considering HRT because you are feeling pretty rough, and a risk of short term side effects for a long term solution is worth braving. If you suffer badly from any of the side effects, you could consider changing the type of HRT you are using. For example, if you struggle with nausea or other digestive problems on oral HRT, you could consider changing to patches.

Remember you are likely to be taking HRT for some time, and your body will need to adjust, so problems are more likely in the early days. Be patient. The long term outcome may well be worth it.

Bleeding

When you first start HRT you may experience some irregular bleeding. This is normal, but if you are concerned you should consult your doctor. Problems with bleeding should settle down after six months.

If after six months you experience any bleeding during your monthly or three monthly combined HRT regime, other than an expected bleed, you should seek advice immediately. In the UK you will find yourself being referred urgently to your local hospital for investigations, including an ultrasound scan, which allows the doctor to visualise the lining of the womb, to check its thickness, and identify polyps, fibroids or anything else that is growing. They may also want to take a small piece of tissue which can be checked for the presence of malignant (cancerous) cells. This may all seem very alarming, but there are a number of possible causes of bleeding, such as the presence of polyps, small benign growths in the lining of the womb, fibroids, or bleeding from the cervix. All of these can be identified and dealt with, and all are far more common than endometrial cancer. The reason for the urgency is that, in the unlikely event that you do have cancer, the problem can be dealt with as quickly as possible.

Ovarian Tissue Freezing

Recently a private company in the UK has been promoting the idea that women should have tissue removed from their ovaries before the menopause kicks in, in fact, the earlier the better. The idea is that this tissue would be transplanted, either to restore fertility, or to delay the menopause by acting as a kind of physiological HRT. Small strips of tissue are removed and frozen, and either put back near the site of the ovary if there is an intention to restore fertility, or in the armpit, if the idea is to delay the menopause. These techniques have been used successfully in pre-menopausal patients who have been treated for cancer, but, as yet, there is no data on their use in menopausal women. At the time of writing, 9 patients have had tissue frozen through this company, for a variety of reasons, and none have yet had them transplanted during a natural menopause.

If it works for cancer patients, why shouldn't it work in healthy older women?

When it comes to delaying, or relieving the symptoms of, the menopause, it may work. However, any relief from menopausal symptoms are unlikely to kick in until a couple of months after the transplant. It does take a few weeks for conventional HRT to become effective, but transplants take longer. It is also important to understand that the transplant has a limited functional life. There have been reports of tissue functioning for as long as 10 years, but they may only survive for one or two years. If you have stored enough tissue you may be able to have repeat transplants each time one fails.

Advocates will tell you that the great advantage of this process is that you will be receiving your own naturally produced hormones from your own tissue, rather than a pharmaceutically prepared product.

On the other hand, HRT has a track record, and is continually improving. It does not involve you spending thousands of pounds or dollars to have surgery (which carries its own risks), store your tissue, and then have it transplanted.

It is also the case that delaying the menopause carries risks, including an increased incidence of breast cancer. If you are hoping for continuing fertility, you should bear in mind that the longer you go on ovulating, the higher your risk of ovarian cancer and, of course, you will go on having periods.

At the moment this is undoubtedly an unproven, experimental technique, and, on that basis, you really should not be paying for it, because no one is in a position to promise you results

Cancer

Cancer is a general term for growth of cells in an abnormal way.

Why do cells grow abnormally?

All the cells in your body contain the same genetic material. Cells are programmed to form particular types of tissue, such as liver, muscle, nerves, or blood, by switching specific genes on or off. This programming also determines how rapidly, and where they grow. Occasionally this programming goes wrong, and cells do not specialise as they should, but continue to grow rapidly as non-specific, or even a completely different type of cell. Wherever cells are growing rapidly or continuously, there is a higher risk of something going wrong, rather like the rate of error in a mass manufacturing process. One of the reasons why exposure to the sun and sunburn increase the risk of skin cancer, is that the skin is repeatedly being damaged and having to repair itself.

The increased risk of endometrial cancer with oestrogen only HRT, occurs because the cells of the endometrium are repeatedly multiplying without being regularly shed, and this constant growth leads to a higher chance of some of the cells losing their identity and starting to grow and multiply abnormally.

Many forms of cancer can now be treated successfully, especially if they are caught early, so it is vital that you report any concerns or warning signs to your doctor.

Chapter 5 - Health after the menopause

Once you have been through the menopause your body should settle down into its post-menopausal state. The symptoms of the menopause will have passed (whether suppressed by HRT, or just naturally diminished). However, your new, oestrogen poor hormone profile presents its own problems.

Osteoporosis

Osteoporosis is one of the conditions most strongly associated with life after the menopause.

Bone is living tissue, just like any other part of the body, and it is constantly renewed and repaired. Most people (it is to be hoped!) only see bone when it is very dead, and only the brittle matrix survives. In life our bones have their own blood supply and are constantly being remodeled. This is because our bones provide the body with a reservoir of calcium. Demand for calcium leads to bones giving up some material, while exercise, and stress on our bones, results in them being built up. Loss of calcium from the bones is controlled by cells called osteoclasts, and is known as bone resorption, while the process of bone formation is controlled by other cells called osteoblasts, and is known as ossification. As a result of this process of bone "remodeling", most of the adult skeleton is renewed every 10 years.

Osteoporosis results when there is more resorption than ossification and the bones are weakened by the loss of calcium, resulting in a high risk of fracture.

Oestrogen inhibits the breakdown of bone through resorption, and may also stimulate bone formation. The drop in oestrogen that occurs at the menopause increases the risk of osteoporosis and fracture. Older women are at higher risk of osteoporosis than men because older men may have higher circulating levels of oestrogen than women.

According to the International Osteoporosis foundation, osteoporosis is estimated to affect 200 million women worldwide - approximately one-tenth of women aged 60, one-fifth of women aged 70, two-fifths of women aged 80 and two-thirds of women aged 90. While that's a lot of women, these figures also tell you that osteoporosis is not inevitable. That is, not everyone gets it. HRT obviously reduces the risk considerably. But there are life style factors that may also impact on your risk of fractures.

OSTEOPOROSIS

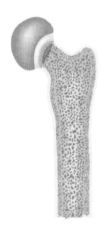
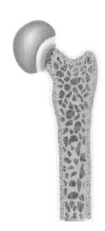

Normal Bone   Bone with Osteoporosis

Risk factors

Women of Caucasian or Asian origin are more at risk, as are lighter thinner women. Having insufficient calcium or vitamin D in your diet will also increase the risk.

Smoking also increases your risk of osteoporosis. I imagine that there are few people who still need convincing that smoking is bad for your health, but you can add this to the list of evils. The picture with regard to alcohol is not quite so clear. There is some evidence that low alcohol consumption, around the single glass a day level, may reduce the risk of fracture, where as high alcohol consumption increases your risk of osteoporosis.

A sedentary lifestyle also increases your risk.

How to reduce your Risk

HRT

Like all other post-menopausal symptoms, HRT will give you some protection from osteoporosis by putting oestrogen back into your system. However, most women take HRT for a limited time during and immediately after the menopause. Eventually you will want to stop taking it, and then your risk of osteoporosis will rise again.

Diet – Calcium

It's fairly obvious that you need to take in calcium in order to maintain the strength of your bones – after all, calcium is the major constituent of the mineral component of bone.

Make sure your diet contains at least the recommended amounts of calcium, so that it is always available when required for bone growth.

The following are good sources of calcium:-

- milk, cheese and other dairy foods.

- green leafy vegetables, such as broccoli, cabbage and okra, but not spinach.

- soya beans.

- tofu.

- soya drinks with added calcium.

- nuts.

- bread and anything made with fortified flour.

- Fish such as sardines and pilchards, where the bones are eaten

Of course you can take calcium supplements but, since vegetables and dairy products form part of a balanced diet, it is always better to get as much as you can through your normal food intake.

Diet – vitamin D

Vitamin D is essential for the absorption of calcium. A lack of vitamin D will inhibit the strengthening and growth of bone. We make our own vitamin D from sunlight. In theory 10-15 minutes of sunlight twice a week would be enough for us to make sufficient vitamin D for healthy bones (and all the other essential functions that require vitamin D). There are two problems with relying on sunlight. We are constantly being reminded not to go out in the sun without sunscreen, and sunscreen would also prevent vitamin D production. Secondly there are parts of the world where we cannot rely on the weather to provide enough sunlight, even in summer. As a result, we need to make sure we have sufficient vitamin D in our diets to compensate. Vitamin D can be obtained from the following foods:-

- oily fish – such as salmon, sardines, herring, mackerel and fresh tuna

- red meat

- liver

- egg yolks

- foods such as most fat spreads and some breakfast cereals, that have been deliberately supplemented with vitamin D

You can also take vitamin D supplements (see also appendix 3), but beware. You can have too much vitamin D. Stick to the recommended levels, and take supplements according to the manufacturer's instructions and you should be fine. If you are concerned about your vitamin D levels, check with your doctor before taking a higher than recommended dose. Too much vitamin D can lead to excessive levels of calcium in the blood. Calcium will then wind up being deposited in various tissues of the body where it doesn't belong, including the kidneys, and this is potentially dangerous.

Exercise

To reduce the risk of bone loss you need high impact, weight bearing exercise. This is not nearly as tough as it sounds. Every time you climb a flight of stairs you are undergoing high impact, weight bearing exercise. As you climb the stairs you are lifting your own weight over and over again, and then taking the impact of your own weight as your feet hit the stairs.

Other high impact weight bearing exercises include dancing, aerobics, jogging and running, tennis, soccer, hockey and hill walking/walking over rough terrain. Just walking is better than nothing, but not nearly as good as if you include some climbing – there is real benefit to lifting your own weight.

How does this help to reduce the risk of osteoporosis and fracture? The action of muscles pulling on bones stimulates the laying down of bone tissue to strengthen the bones. The more exercise you do, the stronger your bones will become.

Generally, in terms of health and longevity, being smaller and lighter is an advantage, but not when it comes to bone strength. Being underweight puts less strain on muscle and bone, and the stimulation of bone growth is reduced.

The advantages of being underweight still outweigh the disadvantages, and you can compensate for being light by exercising using weights. Wrist and ankle weights will help to build up strength, as well as any form of general weight training.

Ideally you should combine a healthy diet with weight bearing exercise – don't rely on one or the other. Supplements should always be a last resort.

Hypertension/High Blood Pressure

Hypertension is one of those conditions strongly associated with the stress of modern life. Interestingly, were you to monitor your blood pressure at times when you consider yourself to be highly stressed, you will probably not see a difference provided you are healthy, and have never suffered from high blood pressure.

There is an association between hypertension and the menopause, but this, like other post-menopausal health issues, is not inevitable, and your personal risk will depend on your general health, and whether you have any history of hypertension.

As we pass the menopause, and with age in general, our body composition shifts. The ratio of lean tissue to fat tissue shifts in favour of fat, and overall there is a trend towards an increased body mass index as we get older. Increased weight and body fat increase the risk of hypertension. However, the real problem is, once more, the drop in oestrogen. Up until the menopause, men are more likely to suffer from hypertension than women. Post-menopausal women catch up and over take the men even when matched for age and body mass index.

What exactly is hypertension?

To function normally we need our blood to flow freely around the body, and for our heart and circulation to respond at times of increased demand, such as during exercise, or at times of stress. This depends on our blood vessels being elastic enough to respond to higher volumes of blood being pumped though the system, and free of any obstructions caused by damage, or the buildup of fatty deposits.

Hypertension (see appendix 4), or raised blood pressure results when the blood vessels are too rigid, obstructed or constricted to allow the blood to flow freely, and pressure builds up. Constant high pressure causes the walls of the arteries to thicken, narrowing the space for the blood to pass through, which in turn raises pressure. High pressure also increases the risk of weak blood vessels bursting, causing serious, potentially fatal blood loss. Narrower blood vessels have higher risk of becoming blocked, and blocked blood vessels can result in vital organs, such as the brain or heart, being starved of blood, leading to a stroke or heart attack.

Oestrogen plays a role in protecting us from the perils of raised blood pressure. It not only helps blood vessels to expand by increasing nitric oxide levels, it also helps reduce the levels of endothelin, a substance that constricts blood vessels and is closely linked to heart disease and high blood pressure.

Collagen and elastin are the main proteins involved in the flexibility and elasticity of tissues including the walls of blood vessels, and their formation is promoted by oestrogen. This flexibility and elasticity are important in enabling the blood vessels to respond to changes in pressure and flow. Rigid blood vessels may be unable to meet demands from the heart.

Oestrogen may also help reduce sodium sensitivity, making women less sensitive to the hypertensive effects of salt. Having too much salt in the blood causes the body to retain water so that the concentration of salt in the blood is kept down. As a result, the volume of blood is increased, and high blood pressure results.

Oestrogen also suppresses the production of substances that trigger the fight-or-flight response that constricts blood vessels, increases heart rate and raises blood pressure.

So with less oestrogen our blood vessels are less flexible, less able to respond to changes in pressure, we are more likely to have increased blood pressure in response to an intake of sodium, and we are more likely to have a fight or flight panic response, which will put a strain on our cardio-vascular system…none of which is good.

The other factor that impacts on your blood pressure and cardiovascular system is insulin resistance. Most people will be aware that insulin, another hormone, is involved in the control of glucose in our blood and in our cells. Many of us will know someone who has to inject insulin in order to keep diabetes under control. Oestrogen facilitates the function of insulin and helps to keep blood sugar levels under control. When oestrogen levels drop we are at greater risk of insulin resistance, in other words, reduced insulin function and higher blood sugar levels. Raised blood sugar puts you at higher risk of hypertension and other cardiovascular problems.

How do I know if I have hypertension?

Unless you have your blood pressure measured, you don't. Hypertension has been called the silent killer because you may be completely unaware of the problem until the consequences become catastrophic.

Hypertension, especially if it is exacerbated by lifestyle factors, just creeps up on you.

So what is your real risk as you pass the menopause? And why is it that despite all these problems women still tend to live longer than men?

30 to 50% of women develop hypertension by the age of 60. The incidence varies with ethnic and socio-economic background, and lifestyle factors naturally play a major part. However, there are highly effective treatments for high blood pressure, and it only becomes life-threatening if it remains untreated, particularly if exacerbated by smoking, drinking, obesity, lack of exercise, and all the other factors that contribute to an unhealthy cardiovascular system. In other words, if you take care of yourself and make an effort to manage your health, you can live with hypertension. To keep your risk of hypertension to a minimum you should:-

- Have your blood pressure checked regularly

- Maintain a healthy weight – obesity in itself may be a cause of hypertension

- Eat heart-healthy foods, such as whole grains, fruits and vegetables.

- Reduce the amount of processed foods and salt in your diet.

- Exercise most days of the week.

- Manage stress.

- Limit or avoid alcohol.

- If you smoke, stop.

Avoid adding salt to food, or buying processed food with a lot of salt added. The daily recommended intake of salt for an adult is 6gms. This is about a teaspoon, so you should check the salt content of your shopping with this figure in mind. Most processed food has salt added, not just for flavour, but because of its preservative action, and so salt levels tend to be high.

Does HRT cause an increase in blood pressure?

There is a general view that anyone on HRT should keep a close eye on their blood pressure, as HRT contains oestrogen, and taking oestrogen can cause hypertension. You will have spotted the contradiction here. If the decrease in oestrogen levels due to the menopause increases the risk of hypertension, how can boosting your oestrogen levels can also cause it?

The answer is that it does not. This myth has its origins in concerns about the contraceptive pill. The oestrogen dose in the Pill is 4 to 10 times more potent than in HRT, and has a different function – it is intended to stop normal reproductive function. The oestrogen in HRT is only intended to put you back to your pre-menopausal levels. High levels of oestrogen can lead to fluid retention which can cause blood pressure to be raised. The strength of the oestrogen in HRT is nowhere near the level required to do this.

If you are on HRT and your blood pressure is raised, make sure you doctor looks for other causes, such as an increase in weight, the possible development of diabetes, or other lifestyle and age linked possibilities. By suspecting your HRT, they may miss the real underlying cause.

HRT does not halt aging, it just deals with the oestrogen related effects of the menopause. There are many other aspects of aging in men and women that may lead to hypertension, including changes in the distribution of body fat, and decreasing amounts of exercise related to problems with aging joints (and weight again).

Heart disease

For the same reasons that the risk of hypertension increases after the menopause, the risk of a cardiovascular "incident" is also higher. "Incident" is a term that encompasses everything from stroke to a heart attack. Adding to the potential for changes in blood pressure, the way we process fats, cholesterol in particular, changes, increasing the risk of fatty deposits building up in our arteries.

Cholesterol

We need cholesterol. It is vital in maintaining the fluidity of our cell membranes, which control how chemicals enter and leave our cells. It is a major component of bile, which is produced in the liver, stored in the gall bladder, and is necessary for the digestion of fat. It is also one of the building blocks of many hormones including oestrogen. Cholesterol becomes more of a hazard to women after our oestrogen levels drop.

In fact, it is not cholesterol itself that is the problem, but the carrier molecules that transport it around the body. There are two types of proteins that transport cholesterol around the body – high density lipoprotein (HDL), and low density lipoprotein (LDL), and we refer to cholesterol carried by HDL as "good" cholesterol, and that carried by LDL as "bad" cholesterol. This is because LDL can build up in the walls of the arteries and cause them to become narrowed or blocked.

Until we reach the menopause we make more "good" cholesterol than "bad" cholesterol. As the influence of oestrogen declines, this reverses and we begin to make more "bad" cholesterol. This increases the risk of fat clogging up our arteries. It also changes in the way fat is deposited around the body, which is why there is an association between a thicker waistline, and (bad) cholesterol levels.

If fat clogs the blood vessels that supply oxygenated blood to the heart, a heart attack will result.

What can we do to reduce our risk of coronary heart disease?

Aside from maintaining oestrogen levels using HRT, our old friends, diet and exercise, are crucial in protecting us from the risk of heart attack.

In terms of diet, the usual suspects, plenty of fruit and vegetables, unsalted nuts, oily fish and olive oil are good sources of unsaturated fats, which provide you with the healthy fat you need to build cell membranes, and for other bodily functions.

On the other hand, you should limit your intake of saturated fats, the kind found in fatty meat and dairy products. This will push up your "bad" cholesterol levels.

However, worse than saturated fats are trans fats. These are found in in some vegetable oils, many baked goods, and some margarine. They occur in small quantities in nature, but it is the manufactured form of trans fats that are the most significant form when it comes to health and disease. While natural saturated fats do contribute some "good" cholesterol, nothing good comes from trans fats, which contribute only "bad" cholesterol. Trans fats are also thought to linked to other health risks, including an increased risk of diabetes, Alzheimer's, depression and behavioural changes. These risks are taken so seriously that some countries have issued guidance about the use of trans fats, regulations limiting their use, or even laws attempting to ban or limit their use.

Sugar

Keep your sugar intake down. Sucrose, the form of sugar that we consume the most of, is made up of glucose, which is essential for life, and fructose, which is not. Only the liver can metabolise fructose. The liver converts fructose to fat, which is released into the blood stream, adding to the body's fat content, and the risk of fat being deposited in blood vessels.

Alcohol

If you are worried about heart disease, but also like a drink or two, you may have read about the phenols contained in red wine, specifically resveratrol, which have antioxidant properties. Consumers of red wine (in moderation) are thought to have lower levels of heart disease, and resveratrol was proposed as the magic ingredient. However, there is no hard evidence that red wine or resveratrol have any real health benefits. Most of the evidence comes from non-human species and has not been replicated in humans. On the other hand, the mythology about the health benefits of red wine is of longstanding, so health conscious people tend to choose it as their drink of choice. The association between red wine and health may not be because red wine makes you healthy, but rather because healthy people drink red wine.

Like so many things that we consume, there are regular and contradictory reports of the effect of alcohol on health. Unless you have been specifically told to avoid it, the occasional drink is unlikely to do much harm, but consider it carefully in combination with other lifestyle factors, and never over indulge.

Your skin after the menopause

Oestrogen is involved in the growth, healing and general physiology of the skin. As levels decline, the skin becomes thinner and loses its elasticity, which results in the formation of wrinkles, and a tendency for the skin to become drier. Oestrogen is also involved in moderating the deposits of fat that support the skin, as well as the circulation that keeps the skin hydrated. Loss of these fat deposits as oestrogen declines, and dehydration due to reduced circulation also contribute to the sagging of the skin.

HRT inevitably delays this to some degree, but there are other measures we can take to slow down the changes in our skin.

Our skin is exposed to assault from both our external and internal environment, and these will affect the speed with which our skin ages. Aside from chronological aging, which is largely determined by genetics, the skin suffers from photo-aging. Exposure to the sun not only increases the risk of skin cancer, it also causes damage that gives the skin a prematurely aged appearance. Not many women aspire to the weather beaten look, so favoured by fictional farmers and fishermen. Ultra-violet light rays have a detrimental effect on the components of skin that give the skin its elasticity. The underlying cause of this is the action of reactive oxygen species, also known as oxygen free radicals (see appendix 5, the antioxidant story). These are highly unstable and reactive forms of oxygen. When they combine with components of our cells and tissues, they change their structure, and damage their potential to function. Not only do they damage cell membranes and proteins, there is the potential for damage to DNA, and more sinister changes, such as those that lead to cancer.

Chronological aging is hard to combat, but photo-aging is something that we can protect ourselves against. You cannot undo the damage that has been done, but you can prevent further damage by avoiding too much direct exposure to the sun, and using a sunscreen with a high protection factor if you must be in the sun. Never go near a sun bed. An artificial tan is certainly not healthy. Tanning beds expose you to concentrated UV rays at close range, much more dangerous than periodic exposure to the sun.

Another avoidable source of free radicals is smoking. Smoking is bad for your health generally, but you may not have considered that it might affect your skin. Cigarette smoke contains carbon monoxide, which displaces the oxygen in your skin, and nicotine, which reduces blood flow, leaving skin dry and discoloured. Cigarette smoking also depletes many nutrients, including vitamin C, which helps to protect against damage by free radicals.

There are so many good reasons not to smoke, and this is just another.

Dehydration is part of skin aging. The changing structure of our skin makes it harder to retain water, so try and avoid anything that might exacerbate this. Alcohol and caffeine dehydrate our systems generally, so if you must indulge, try to limit your consumption, or at least make sure you drink plenty of water to compensate.

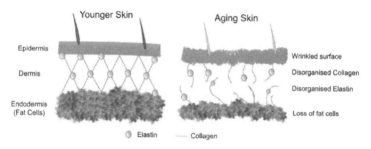

Can cosmetic creams stop or reduce wrinkles and other forms of skin aging?

Sadly, there are no over the counter products that will stop or reverse the aging process. However, moisturisers will help to keep your skin hydrated and smooth, which can help to slow down aging. Certainly letting your skin dry out can accelerate the aging process.

The main types of moisturisers are:

Humectants

These contain molecules that attract water from lower layers of the skin into the surface layers. There are both synthetic and natural humectants. Synthetic humectants will act to draw up moisture but do not add anything back into the skin. Glycerin is one of the main ingredients in these types of preparation but this tends to give the cream a tacky, greasy texture. Natural humectants include honey, hyaluronic acid, and aloe vera. Aloe vera has become something of a health cult, with claims that it will sooth everything from acne to hot flushes, to irritable bowel syndrome. The evidence for most of these claims is largely anecdotal, but there is no doubt that aloe vera gel will help to keep your skin hydrated, and is non greasy, so will not make things worse for those with oily skin.

Occlusives

Occlusives prevent moisture from evaporating from the skin surface. They are made up of agents that do not mix with water, and therefore block water from passing through. By nature, these tend to be oily or waxy. A moisturiser that consists of an occlusive alone is likely to be heavy and greasy – the sort of cream you might want to put on in the depths of winter, but not during more temperate times.

Emollients

These act on flaky surface cells to smooth them out. They also have occlusive activity, and form a layer over the surface of the skin to limit evaporation.

Most cosmetic moisturisers contain a mixture of these types of ingredients, as well as other chemicals that may colour or add scent. Try to avoid perfumed creams as these add no value in terms of the health of your skin, and may actually have a drying effect.

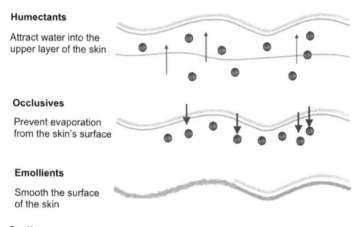

Humectants

Attract water into the upper layer of the skin

Occlusives

Prevent evaporation from the skin's surface

Emollients

Smooth the surface of the skin

Collagen creams

Some "anti-aging" creams contain collagen, one of the molecules that gives our skin its elasticity, and which breaks down with age. Sadly, the skin cannot absorb collagen from creams. It is a very large molecule, and the skin is a pretty effective barrier against even small molecules, such as water, so there is no way in for something the size of collagen. Any effect of creams containing collagens has more to do with superficially filling wrinkles on a temporary basis.

Taking collagen as a dietary supplement will not work either. Collagen is assembled in the skin from smaller molecules. There is no way for a fully formed collagen molecule to make its way into the structure of your skin.

In fact, anything that enters the body and changes the way it works, or its structure would no longer be a cosmetic, but a drug, and you would not be able to pick it up in your super market. Whether the claims are for collagen, or penta-peptides, or any other ingredient, nothing that you buy over the counter will get rid of your wrinkles, or stop them forming.

My skin cream makes my face tingle so it must be doing something...

If your face tingles when you use a particular product it is usually because it contains a mild acid that is added exfoliator, i.e. it will burn dead cells from the surface of the skin. You should adjust to this if you continue using it, but it really is not a good idea to treat your skin so harshly, especially as it is beginning to age.

Nothing will permanently tighten the skin, or remove wrinkles except cosmetic surgery, a measure to be taken only in desperation.

Other creams claim to form or tighten the skin. Skin tightening preparations may make your skin tingle and give you a (temporary) healthy glow. This is done by drying out the skin, using astringent chemicals, which is not good for aging skin in the long term.

Stick to moisturisers, keeping them as simple as possible, protect your skin from the sun, smoke, and other pollutants, drink plenty of water and keep to a healthy diet.

Think of your skin in terms of its health rather than trying to be eternally youthful. Your overall health will do more for your skin than a sack full of cosmetics.

What are age spots?

Oestrogen is involved in controlling production of the skin pigment, melanin, by specific skin cells known as melanocytes. The pigment is produced to protect our skin when it is exposed to the sun. As we age and oestrogen declines, the production of melanin is less well controlled, and it may be produced in excess, especially in areas of the skin exposed to the sun. The dark patches that result are known as age spots, or liver spots, or, more formally, solar lentigines. They are normal, and harmless, and do not turn into cancerous moles, or melanomas. However, it is not always easy to tell the difference between an age spot and a potentially cancerous mole. If you are at all concerned you should consult your doctor.

Age spots are not pretty, but generally they only bother us because they remind us we are getting older. You can have them removed using laser treatment, or cryosurgery/therapy, which involves killing the pigmented cells by freezing them. There are other chemical and abrasive techniques for removing the layer of dark cells. However, if they are not unsightly, and don't bother you, leave them well alone. The use of sunscreens can help to prevent more forming, especially on the face, which is, of course, exposed more than any other part of your skin.

Your Hair after the Menopause

As your hormone levels change with the menopause, you may notice changes in your hair. You may find that your hair and scalp tend to be dry. You may also notice that you are shedding more hair than usual as you go through the menopause, but this will probably settle down once your hormone levels stop changing.

Going grey

Most women start noticing grey hairs around the age of 35. The menopause does not accelerate this. It happens at a fairly steady rate, and fifty percent of people have fifty percent grey hair by the age of fifty.

Female pattern baldness

Female pattern baldness is quite different to male pattern baldness, as it involves thinning and loss of hair all over the head. It has a significant genetic component, so if either of your parents suffered significant hair loss, your risk will be higher. Oestrogen prevents hair follicles from shrinking and from stopping producing hair. When oestrogen levels drop, the influence of testosterone becomes more significant, and those hair follicles that are genetically disposed to this condition shrink and produce thinner hair fibres that are more likely to break. Ultimately these follicles will stop producing hair altogether. If you are concerned about hair loss, it is better to seek help sooner rather than later. There are treatments available that promote regrowth of hair. As this is considered to be a cosmetic problem, you may well have to pay for any treatment.

If you seem to be losing hair suddenly and dramatically consult your doctor immediately, as this may be a symptom of some serious problem.

On the other hand, while the majority of women will experience some hair loss by the time they are over 70, it is a gradual, not a dramatic process.

As usual, a healthy lifestyle (especially one that avoids stress), will help to promote the health of your hair.

Dental Health

During or after the menopause you may notice changes in your gums. Gum recession is common, and this means we need to pay more attention to our dental health to prevent infection and gum disease that could increase the loss of gum tissues, and tooth decay.

In severe cases, osteoporosis can affect the jaw, causing teeth to loosen or be lost.

For most women with a healthy diet and lifestyle, a good dental hygiene routine will enable you to keep your teeth into old age. Make sure you keep up your regular visit to the dentist and the hygienist, and follow any advice they may give you.

Eye Health

Post-menopausal women are more likely to develop cataracts that men of the same age. This is apparently the only age related condition that carries a higher risk for women than men.

The lenses in our eyes are made of protein and water, arranged to form a clear, glass like structure. As a we age, the protein may begin to clump together, forming cloudy areas in the lens. The precise reason why this occurs is not known, but a number of risk factors have been identified. It probably will not surprise you to read that smoking, drinking, and exposure to sunlight can all increase your risk of developing cataracts and the speed at which they develop. Obesity and hypertension are also associated with an increased risk.

When it comes to cataracts HRT has a mixed press. Initially it was thought that HRT was associated with an increased risk of cataracts, but more recent studies suggest that the oestrogen in HRT actually has a protective effect, and actually helps to decrease the risk.

What are the symptoms of cataracts?

Cloudy/Blurry vision

Faded colours

Glare – lights, and sunlight may seem too bright, and a halo may appear around lights.

Reduced night vision

Double vision

If you are experiencing any of these, however minor, you should get your eyes checked.

Can I reduce the risk?

One theory is that the lenses are affected by oxidative changes in the proteins, in other words, those free radicals may have a role in this too. Eating a diet high in fruit and vegetables, which have a high anti-oxidant content may help to reduce your risk. In fact, research has shown this to be the case, although "eye vitamins" and "vision supplements" do not appear to have any effect. For some reason, anti-oxidants need to be acquired naturally from the diet to have an effect.

Generally, as you move into the post-menopausal phase, you should be aware of your eyes, as well as the rest of your health. Make sure you have regular tests, so that any conditions can be identified and dealt with as early as possible.

Sex after the Menopause

There is no reason why you should not continue to have an enjoyable sex life after the menopause. It has been said that the brain is our primary sexual organ. It coordinates all the factors that lead to sexual arousal, including sights, smells, sounds, and even memories. These don't stop working just because our oestrogen levels have fallen. Some women are more relaxed about sex after the menopause, because they are no longer concerned about the risk of pregnancy.

On the other hand, you may find that you are less interested in sex, and arousal happens less easily than before the menopause. How negatively this affects you depends in part on whether you have a partner, and how they feel about it. Otherwise it is fine to be less interested in sex.

If you are interested, you may find there are problems with physical arousal.

Vaginal dryness, which results from the drop in oestrogen, especially if you are not using HRT, may be generally uncomfortable, but is a serious issue when it comes to sex, and can result in dyspareunia (pain on intercourse). To deal with this your doctor may prescribe local oestrogen treatment in the form of creams, pessaries or vaginal rings. This is like having HRT applied directly to the vagina, to stop the cells of the vagina from shutting down, and to promote the production of the natural lubricants that are produced in response to sexual arousal.

For this to work oestrogen must be absorbed into the cells, and it is inevitable that some reaches the blood stream.

So do these oestrogen preparations carry the same kind of risks as HRT taken by mouth?

Because oestrogen is being applied directly to the area where the effect is needed, much lower doses are needed than for oral HRT. Oral doses are measured in milligrams, while local doses are in micrograms (1/1000 milligram). Unless you have a history of breast cancer, which is oestrogen sensitive, or have been experiencing unusual vaginal bleeding there should be no reason why your doctor would not prescribe oestrogen therapy. Your doctor will discuss any risk factors from your medical history, before prescribing oestrogen treatment, as well as the risks and possible side effects. The risks are similar to those of oral HRT, but at a much lower level, because the dose is lower, and there will be comparatively little oestrogen in your circulation.

What is the difference between the creams, pessaries or rings?

Creams must be applied nightly. If you are still using contraception you need to be aware that they may cause damage to condoms or caps/diaphragms. If this is a problem, you should consider using pessaries or the ring.

Pessaries are inserted in the vagina using an applicator supplied with the medication. The usually dose is one per day for the first two weeks, and then one twice a week after that.

The vaginal ring is inserted high into the vagina, and will need replacing approximately every three months. These rings are made of flexible silicon, and once they are in place you should not be able to feel them. In some ways this is the most convenient way to take oestrogen, as you can forget about it most of the time.

In all cases your doctor will want to see you regularly to monitor your response, and it may be weeks or even months before you feel the full effects.

Your doctor is unlikely to continue to prescribe oestrogen therapy indefinitely, as any risks may increase with the length of time the medication is used.

If you would rather avoid any form of HRT, then you could try using over the counter vaginal lubricants from your local pharmacy. You may want to use these in any case, while you wait for your oestrogen therapy to take full effect.

Bear in mind that, if you have an understanding partner, there are many ways of having a satisfying physical relationship without penetrative sex.

Chapter 6 - Fertility after the menopause

Why reproduction just can't happen..

For women hoping to conceive from their mid-forties onwards, the statistics do not make encouraging reading. By the age of 45 your chance of conceiving naturally is around 1%. The chance of miscarriage if you do get pregnant is about 50%, and your chance of having a child with Downs syndrome is 1 in 30.

Although your ovaries finally shut down at the time of the menopause, they will have been in semi-retirement for some time before that. Even while you are still having periods, your reserve of eggs is more or less exhausted – and any eggs that you do have carry a high risk of being chromosomally abnormal, which is why the odds of having a child with Down's syndrome, which is caused by having an extra copy of chromosome 21, is increased.

The reason eggs become increasingly abnormal with age, lies in their origin before we are born. At birth our ovaries contain all the eggs we will ever have. They underwent a series of complex divisions while we were still in the womb, so that they are ready for the final stage of development that happens at the time of ovulation. It seems that the mechanism of division becomes less efficient the longer the cell has been waiting in this state. By the time we have lived five decades, those chromosomes have been poised for division for a very long time, and the result is a high chance of error, a high chance that the chromosomes will divide in an abnormal way. Some of these abnormalities lead to miscarriage, because the embryos that form are too abnormal to survive. Apart from miscarriage, and the higher chance of Down's syndrome, there are other conditions associated with pregnancies in later life, some more severe than Down's, some less, all associated with the way chromosomes divide and interact.

After the menopause, not only have you the problem of having only a few, possibly abnormal eggs, but you will have stopped producing the hormones that induce ovulation, prepare the lining of the womb, and support a pregnancy.

There are some rare records of natural pregnancies in women over 50 - the two oldest natural mothers were both on HRT at the time, but it is as reasonable to presume that you will not get pregnant once you reach the menopause as it is to assume that the lottery ticket you have bought will not be a winner (the chance of any one ticket being a winner in the UK national lottery is 1 in 14 million).

If it is so difficult to conceive once you reach your mid-forties, how is it that we read about so many celebrities who have babies later in life?

The fact is that the majority of women who conceive at 45 plus, have had more than a little help. They have had in-vitro fertilization treatment using eggs donated by a younger woman, usually under 35, who may have had her own family, and so has proven fertility.

Once you have a fertilized egg, all you have to do is prepare the lining of the womb, and maintain the pregnancy. This can be done using a form of HRT – and this means that it is possible to become pregnant, not only in your late forties, but after the menopause. Assuming you still have your womb, it should be capable of responding to exogenous (from the outside) hormones, given as tablet, or injections. Eggs from a donor may be fertilised by sperm from your partner if you have a male partner, or from a donor if you do not. They develop into embryos in the laboratory, and then one or two would be placed in your womb, where a nice thick, hormonally prepared lining awaits them. Simple – well not really. The process may cost thousands of pounds, and there is no guarantee of success – and then there are other problems.

These can be divided into the risks of pregnancy at an advanced age, and the problems associated with donated eggs.

The risks of post-menopausal pregnancy

While the use of donated eggs reduces the risk of chromosomal abnormalities down to the risk associated with the donor's age, there are a number of potential physical problems for both mothers and children.

Pregnancy at any age carries a number of health risks, hypertension (high blood pressure), diabetes induced by pregnancy (gestational diabetes), pre-eclampsia (a condition associated initially with hypertension), and in severe cases, a decline in liver and kidney function, breakdown of red blood cells, fluid in the lungs and seizures), and placenta praevia, a condition where the placenta attaches close to the opening of the neck of the womb. These risks are all higher in older mothers – placenta praevia is particularly associated with older mothers, and the risk of having a premature birth, or of a very low birth weight is also much increased in mothers over 50. While in theory the womb could go on responding to hormones until the day you die, the rest of your body will lose the strength and adaptability that pregnancy requires. Our hearts and circulatory system are put under considerable strain by pregnancy, and a 50 plus year old cardio-vascular system may struggle to sustain two lives.

The problems with donated eggs

You will need to come to terms with the fact that your child will not be genetically related to you. Research has shown that women find this easier to deal with than infertile men, whose partners have children with donated sperm This is not surprising as women still have the experience of pregnancy and of giving birth and are likely to feel a bond with the child because of this. In the UK, centres offering treatment with donated eggs are likely to insist on your having counselling so that you can talk through all the implications of treatment.

In the past we would have accepted the inevitability of our biology. If you did not succeed in conceiving in your twenties of thirties, or, indeed, did not have the opportunity, you would have accepted that pregnancy was something you simply would not experience. These days, in the face of medical advances, our expectations are different. If you meet the one you want to have children with after your ovaries have shut down, pregnancy is no longer impossible. It may be that you have simply not been in a position, either financially, or because of other commitments, to care for a child. For many women it would seem that middle age is the ideal time. They are better off, have more time, more patience and experience. All this has to be weighed against the health risks, the costs, the complexities, and the fact that you will have less time left to spend with your children, although with the average life expectancy for women in the UK now at 83, this last point is no longer as significant as it once was.

In your fifties you may feel you still have plenty of energy for bringing up a child, but many doctors feel that the risks at 50 plus, are more significant that the benefits. For a medical practitioner this is a difficult call. They will see it very differently to the treatment of a pre-menopausal woman with some pathology that has led to infertility. Those cases represent treatment of a medical condition. There is nothing to treat in women over fifty, since the state of being unable to conceive after the menopause is entirely natural. The fact that the technology exists, doesn't mean that it is reasonable to make it available to anyone and everyone.

In India it has been made available to women in their seventies, with reports of first pregnancies occurring at 70, and 72. These are not spritely 50 year olds, who could pass for 40. These are elderly women in a country where 70 is the average female life expectancy.

Daljinder Kaur gave birth to her son in 2016, when she was 72. Her husband has said that they are not worried about their child's future should they die, because God "will take care of everything."

Just a few weeks ago, as I write this, 74 year-old Erramatti Mangayamma gave birth to twins. Her husband collapsed with a heart attack the day after the birth, and Erramatti has remained in intensive care since undergoing a caesarean section. The babies are apparently healthy and being cared for by relatives.

These are extremes, but they are the ultimate outcome of an approach that says if something is possible, and you want it, then you should have it.

In countries where reproductive technology is regulated, the future of the potential children forms part of the decision making process, and the Hippocratic approach of "first do not harm" may well stop clinical professionals from taking risks with the lives of their patients, however much the patient desires the possible outcome, and is happy to accept the risk.

If you are still determined, sadly there will always be someone prepared to treat you for the right price.

Fertility tourism, the idea of travelling to find a clinic in a country where professionals do not feel constrained by risks or ethics, is a well known phenomenon. At this point we need to consider the donors. Many of us are horrified by the idea that vulnerable people could be paid for donating a kidney, but don't think of egg donation in the same way. While the health risks, although they do exist, are much lower than in live kidney donation, women are being paid to hand over their genetic heritage. In some countries, like the UK, there is a cap on the amount an egg donor can be paid legally. In others, donors may be paid thousands of dollars, and even where rules exist, illegal private deals inevitably take place.

If fate deprived you of the opportunity to experience pregnancy and motherhood at the time when you might have achieved it unaided, you may feel that you are entitled to make up for this by taking advantage of modern medical technology. It is your choice, but it is important to go into it with your eyes wide open, with realistic expectations, and a full understanding of the risks and difficulties you are likely to face – and if you must do it, the sooner the better.

Chapter 7 - The Last Word...

About 20 years ago, I was being wheeled back from the operating theatre after a minor procedure. Seeing that I was awake, the nurse walking beside asked me if I was in any pain. Yes, I told her, quite a lot, not unreasonably thinking she might offer to do something about it. "Oh well", she said, "It's all part of being a woman." This was a rather disturbing perspective from a female, and a member of the caring profession. But it was only a few decades ago that this was a popular view. Women suffered. They suffered to give birth, they suffered on a monthly basis if they were not pregnant, and they suffered through the menopause. Women themselves were largely responsible for propagating this myth, as though suffering made them somehow better people, along the lines of "what does not kill me makes me strong". However, in the second half of the twentieth century, developments in science and medicine lead to a revolution in women's healthcare, and gave women choices that meant that suffering was no longer inevitable. Changes in our approach to all aspects of female health, from childbirth, to contraception, to HRT, and an increased understanding of all things hormonal and gynaecological, including why some of us have such painful periods, while others have none at all, have led to greatly improved methods of dealing with the less comfortable aspects of female biology.

Once we have passed the menopause we have much better expectations in terms of quality of continued life. We can choose to avoid the ongoing risks of oestrogen attenuation by taking HRT, or, if we decide that the risks and potential side effects outweigh the discomforts of oestrogen withdrawal, there are other aids, such as oestrogen gels for vaginal dryness, supplements to ward off osteoporosis, not to mention clear lifestyle advice for reducing our risks of hypertension and heart disease.

Good nutrition and good medical care and advice throughout our lives, mean that out life expectancy is greater than ever. We no longer believe that passing into middle age and on into old age means a slowing down, a blue rinse, and a twinset and pearls. We expect to be able to carry on busy active lives, past the menopause, and, for those of us lucky enough to do so, after we retire – and that is the problem with the menopause. It gets in the way of our expectations. It can slow us down, sap our energy, and leave us struggling to maintain a positive outlook. We feel, in the modern world, this should not be happening to us. However, for all our advances, and our technology, we are still animals, and our biology will do what it has always done. You have a choice about the way you deal with it. You can see it off with medication, or focus on maintaining a healthy lifestyle, with a positive outlook, and look forward to the next phase of your life – a life without periods, a life without a need to worry about contraception, a life that can be healthy and happy for many years to come, provided you treat your body and mind with respect.

You have control. The menopause may be inevitable, but armed with knowledge and understanding you need not fear it. You should be facing your sixth decade with optimism, not dread. After all, aging is not just a matter of the physical, it is also cultural. You may have preconceived ideas about aging and changes in expectation and behaviour, but modern health care, and general attitudes have led to the suggestion that 60 is the new 40. Many women reach their peak of achievement in their post-menopausal lives, by changing their focus to something they have never had time to do before. Anna Mary Moses, known to the word as Grandma Moses, took up painting in earnest when she was 78, and her exhibitions broke attendance records. She produced over 1500 works in the last 3 decades of her life. Others, especially those with creative careers, see no reason to stop, just because a chronological landmark has ticked by – look at Vivienne Westwood and Helen Mirren, both icons in their 70s. In other words, the menopause and its legacy is no barrier to achievement or enjoyment of life.

The information in this book should enable you to plan to tackle the menopause, and life beyond it. You may be one of the lucky ones, like my mother, who barely noticed it – or you might be like me, and feel a little ambushed until you have worked out what is happening and instigated your plan for dealing with it. Either way you should not feel threatened by the menopause, any more than you were by adolescence. You are stepping into the third phase of your life, life being the most important word here. After all there's only one way to completely avoid the menopause, and it has very little appeal. In the Western World, women are, on average, expected to live into their early eighties so you may have twenty-five to thirty years or more ahead of you (see appendix 6, Why do women live longer than men?). Thirty years was the average human life expectancy in the eighteenth century, and today it is the length of many people's working lives.

It is up to you. You can face the menopause head on, and tackle the problems as they arise, and remember that this is a temporary phase, that the symptoms will pass, and that research has given us options for relief in the mean time – and you can look forward to the rest of your life. Take a positive attitude and you will find that what might be regarded as "menopausal miseries" become just minor inconveniences in the course of your life.

Useful Contacts

Women's Health Concern – the patient arm of the British Menopause Society http://www.womens-health-concern.org/

Menopause Matters – a great information resource

http://www.menopausematters.co.uk/

Royal College of Obstetrics and Gynaecology – resources on medication and self-care

https://www.rcog.org.uk/en/patients/menopause/

North American Menopause Society – has information for patients as well as professionals

https://www.menopause.org/

Australasian Menopause Society – infographics, factsheets, videos and self-assessment tools for various health risks.

https://www.menopause.org.au/

If you have any questions or comments about this book, please email info@beatthemenopause.com

Appendix 1 - Evidence

In order to assess whether a treatment works, we need to examine the evidence. The best evidence is an independent randomised controlled, double blind clinical trial. The worst evidence is the story of a friend of a friend. The National Institute for Clinical Excellence in the UK assesses the efficacy of treatments based on the quality of the evidence, and recommends therapies on this basis. When making decisions you need to employ a version of this. If something has no evidence to support it, especially if trials have shown no effect, it is unlikely to help you. Beware of studies commissioned or sponsored by the manufacturer. Equally, beware of those who are enthusiastic about particular types of medicine for what amounts to sentimental reasons. We feel that somehow herbal, more natural, remedies should be better than nasty chemicals. Sadly, the nasty chemicals have a far higher chance of succeeding because they have been specifically designed and manufactured to deal with a specific   problem.

In this book the only reason for dismissing a remedy is lack of evidence. St John's Wort is a "natural" or "herbal" remedy, but it has plenty of scientific evidence behind it. If you take something that has no evidence behind it and it works, that's great. You feel better, and that is the most important thing - but remember you are an uncontrolled experiment. It might have happened anyway.

Appendix 2 - CBT

What is CBT?

Cognitive behavioural therapy involves helping patients to understand how their thoughts influence their feelings and behavior. Although principally developed to treat depression and anxiety, it is used to treat a wide range of conditions. In addition to depression or anxiety disorders, CBT can also help people with

- post-traumatic stress disorder (PTSD)

- obsessive compulsive disorder

- panic disorder

- phobias

- eating   disorders –   such as anorexia and bulimia

- sleep problems – such as insomnia

- problems related to alcohol misuse

- CBT is also sometimes used to treat people with long-term health conditions, such as:

- irritable bowel syndrome (IBS)

- chronic fatigue syndrome (CFS)

Although CBT can't cure the physical symptoms of these conditions, it can help people cope better with their symptoms. This is really the only way it could offer any help with hot flushes, by giving patients a coping mechanism.

Appendix 3 - Low Vitamin D and fatigue

Low vitamin D levels have relatively recently been associated with fatigue and general muscle aches. On both sides of the Atlantic it has become fashionable to test for vitamin D levels in cases of chronic fatigue. Vitamin supplement manufacturers are having a wonderful time with this, as you can imagine, but real vitamin D deficiency is rare. Having a low level, and having a real deficiency are not the same thing. If you are going through the menopause you are likely to be experiencing symptoms that might be associated with vitamin D deficiency – but your symptoms are caused by oestrogen deficiency. The reason to consider ensuring that you have enough vitamin D in your system once you are through the menopause, is purely to mitigate against the risk of osteoporosis. If you are suffering from acute fatigue you should consult your doctor before taking anything. If you are going to take a vitamin D supplement you only need 5-10µg per day – you should not take more than 25µg.

Appendix 4 - Why we should watch our blood pressure..

The arteries carry blood from the heart to all the organs and muscles of the body, to give them the energy and oxygen they need. They have muscular walls that allow them to expand or contract in response to different stimuli. Wider arteries let more blood through, narrow, contracted arteries speed up the flow of blood, and also help the body to retain heat.

If blood is constantly being pumped through the arteries at high pressure, the constant pushing against the artery walls may cause damage, or cause the artery walls to thicken in response to constant pressure, which, in turn, may narrow the space in the arteries. High pressure on weakened artery walls may cause them to rupture.

How your arteries affect your blood pressure

High blood pressure can affect the ability of the arteries to open and close. If your blood pressure is too high, the muscles in the artery wall will respond by pushing back harder. This will make them grow bigger, which makes your artery walls thicker.

Thicker arteries mean that there is less space for the blood to flow through. This will raise your blood pressure even further

What happens when your arteries become too narrow?

The higher your blood pressure is, the greater the chance that the extra pressure could make a weak artery burst. Also, the narrower your arteries are, the greater the risk that they could become blocked.

If an artery bursts or becomes blocked, the part of the body that gets its blood from that artery will be starved of the energy and oxygen it needs and the cells in the affected area will die.

If the burst artery supplies a part of the brain, then the result is a stroke. If the burst artery supplies a part of the heart, then that area of heart muscle will die, causing a heart attack.

How you can help your arteries

You can help your arteries to stay healthy by keeping your blood pressure controlled, and by following a healthy lifestyle.

Healthy eating will give your body the energy and nutrients it needs to keep it in good condition. Getting active will also keep your heart and blood vessels fit and healthy.

Many of the medicines used to treat high blood pressure work to keep the arteries wider. They do this by acting directly on the muscles in the artery wall, or by controlling hormones that act on these muscles

What is a stroke?

Uncontrolled high blood pressure can cause problems by damaging and narrowing the blood vessels in your brain. Over time, this raises the risk of a blood vessel becoming blocked or bursting.

If blood cannot carry energy and oxygen to part of the brain due to a blocked or burst blood vessel, some cells in the brain may be damaged, or even die. This is called a stroke, and it can lead to disability and even death.

Appendix 5 - The Anti-Oxidant story

Oxygen is essential for life. Without oxygen to breathe, we die. Oxygen is our source of energy. Oxygen is also an essential component of the molecules that make up our bodies, and control our physiology. Not only do we breathe in oxygen, but we swallow it as a component of sugars, proteins and fats.

It is literally vital stuff.

Like many things that are good for us in just the right quantities too much oxygen, and in particular forms, is bad for us.

Breathing pure oxygen is poisonous if you do it for too long. In any case a pure oxygen atmosphere would be very dangerous as oxygen is highly explosive given the slightest encouragement - but at atmospheric concentrations oxygen gas is not usually a problem. Oxygen gas is made up of molecules consisting of two oxygen atoms. Joined together, oxygen atoms are fairly stable. Split apart, they are not. Oxygen atoms are highly reactive, ready to combine with a variety of other chemicals, to form new compounds that will make them stable again.

Oxygen atoms in a reactive state, either alone, or in combination with other atoms, are known as reactive oxygen species, or oxygen free radicals. They are an essential part of the chemistry of our cells, but these same cells have mechanisms to neutralise excess amounts of free radicals. Under normal circumstances the body copes very well with free radicals.

However, if we are exposed to conditions that cause the level of free radicals to become so high that we can no longer neutralise them, then they have the potential to cause damage to components of our cells. This is known as oxidative stress.

One of the most significant components of our cells, DNA, is vulnerable to damage by free radicals. They can alter the structure of DNA which, in turn, changes the way it functions. Since DNA governs which proteins our cells make and how they behave, such changes may be damaging and even dangerous. Our cells have a continuous programme of DNA repair, but they may not be able to keep it up if the damage is excessive.

Free radical damage has been blamed for everything from wrinkles to cancer. This is entirely understandable given that cancer generally results from abnormal genetic behaviour in cells and this is quite possibly the result of DNA damage.

Excessive free radical generation can be caused by exposure to ultra-violet rays from the sun, smoking, exposure to tobacco smoke, exposure to high levels of atmospheric pollutants, physical and psychological stress and even certain elements of our diets.

What is an anti-oxidant?

Anti-oxidants are molecules that react with free radicals to form new molecules that are stable. They are often referred to as scavengers, because of the way they appear to mop up the free radicals. They are highly reactive molecules themselves, which means that the free radicals are more likely to react with them than with important components of our cells.

In recent years, antioxidant has become the magic word for something that will cure anything from wrinkles to macular degeneration (an eye condition that can lead to blindness). Our increased understanding of the actions of free-radicals, and the need to neutralise them has not gone unnoticed by the world of marketing. A decade or so ago, it might have been unusual to find blueberries in your local supermarket. Since they have been found to contain high levels of anti oxidants, they are everywhere.

Skin creams will claim to have anti-oxidant properties, often in the form of co-enzyme Q10, and health food stores sell a multitude of anti-oxidant dietary supplements.

But do they work?

Anti-oxidant vitamins such as vitamins C and E do seem to give some protection against oxidative damage, especially when taken in combination.

The ARED (age related eye disease) study has shown that regular doses of specific anti oxidants and zinc have significant effects in slowing down age related macular degeneration, and may even prevent its advance altogether.

Blueberries certainly contain a high level of anti-oxidant compounds, but it is not certain that the body can utilise these when you obtain them directly from the fruit. There is, however, some evidence for the use of blueberry extract.

Lycopene, a powerful anti-oxidant which is extracted from tomatoes and found in tomato concentrates, such as soups, has been shown to reduce free-radical induced DNA damage in all types of cells, and is even recommended to men who are concerned about fertility and DNA damage to their sperm.

The polyphenol compounds in green tea are thought to have highly beneficial anti-oxidant properties, but you will need to drink 3 to 5 cups per day to get any health benefits.

Can you absorb anti-oxidants through your skin?

Apparently you can. This is the best way to get vitamins C and E into your skin cells, as they will absorb these at much higher concentrations than would be achieved by taking them by mouth. However, over the counter preparations are unlikely to contain the active forms of these vitamins in sufficient quantities to have an effect, so you are probably better off taking them by mouth.

And Co-enzyme Q10?

Co- enzyme Q10 occurs naturally in the body and definitely has anti-oxidant properties. This does not mean that putting it in a moisturiser will deliver it to the cells that need it. In fact there is no evidence that over the counter products containing this molecule will have any effect existing or future free-radical damage.

Anti oxidants certainly have beneficial effects on health, by limiting the damage done by free radicals, and reducing the risk of oxidative stress. This does not mean that a product that proclaims that it "contains anti-oxidants" is actually going to do you any good.

It would make more sense to ensure that your diet contains a good mix of vitamins and anti-oxidant containing foods – and the nutritionists say, evidence or no evidence, keep eating those blueberries…

Appendix 6 – Why do women live longer than men?

And why do women live longer than men, despite their propensity to hypertension (and cardio-vascular incidents – see below) as they age?

We have plenty of data to show that female children have lower mortality rates than males, and there is also some evidence that females have a genetic advantage, having two X-chromosomes, and therefore two copies of all the genes the X-chromosome carries – in other words, females have a back up – where as males only have the one, and the Y-chromosome which is pretty useless for anything other than conferring maleness. This does not entirely explain the difference in average life expectancy. It now seems likely that different behaviours between males and females play a considerable part in the discrepancy in life expectancy. Life expectancy is usually defined as life expectancy at birth, so if one gender or the other were more likely to die young, the average life expectancy would be lowered. In 2017 in the UK, the average lifespan was 79.2 years for men, and 82.9 for women. This is a fairly small different, but it is significant due to the very large numbers involved. Anthropologically, males are the risk takers, and are generally more likely to be exposed to risk. In modern societies the risks have largely been taken out of obtaining food and protecting the family. However, males are thought to be more pre-disposed to physical risk taking, and more likely to drink and smoke (although the sexes are rapidly converging on all these points). If we take behaviour on the road as an example, in the UK, in percentage terms, twice as many men as women have points for speeding. Even if you correct for time spent driving, and the type of cars driven, there is a difference. In general terms, a propensity for risk taking is likely to shorten your life span. Add to this the fact that women tend to be more conscious of their health and appearance, and more likely to seek and act on medical advice, which is borne out by the fact that there are still more male smokers than female, then it would begin to look as though the difference in lifespan has as much to do with behaviours as it has to do with genetics.

In the UK in 2017, one in five men could expect to live to the age of ninety, compared with one in three women. If they reach ninety men would be likely to have another four years of life, compared with four point six for women. The gap, compared with life expectancy at birth, has narrowed from 3.8 years to just 0.6 years. This suggests that the advantage of being female declines as we grow into extreme old age. What is left might well be the small advantage conferred by genetics and listening to our doctors.

Printed in Great Britain
by Amazon

46715403R00081